THEIR RIGHTS

Advance directives and
living wills explored

Dedication

This book is dedicated to all who helped Kevin Kendrick and me to pull it together: to our longsuffering families and our colleagues.

It is also dedicated to the memory of John and Barbara McKinnon, my late parents in law. They were both doctors and embodied in their work precisely the care for the whole person that is stressed in this book.

It is now also dedicated to the memory of Kevin Kendrick.

Simon Robinson

THEIR RIGHTS

Advance directives and living wills explored

Kevin Kendrick and
Simon Robinson

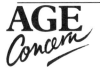

BOOKS

© 2002 Kevin Kendrick and Simon J. Robinson

Published by Age Concern England
1268 London Road
London SW16 4ER

First published 2002

Editor Richenda Milton-Thompson
Design and typesetting GreenGate Publishing Services
Printed in Great Britain

A catalogue record for this book is available from the British Library

ISBN 0–86242–244–2

Bulk orders
Age Concern England is pleased to offer customised editions of all its titles to UK companies, institutions or other organisations wishing to make a bulk purchase. For further information, please contact the Publishing Department at the address on this page. Tel: 020 8765 7200. Fax: 020 8765 7211. Email: books@ace.org.uk

Contents

About the authors

Kevin Kendrick was lecturer in Nursing in the School of Healthcare Studies, University of Leeds from 1997, until his untimely death from a road accident in 2001. He specialised in healthcare ethics, palliative care and spirituality and healthcare. Other books include: *Themes and Perspectives in Nursing; Ethical Counselling - A Workbook for Nurses; Innovations in Nursing Practice.*

Simon J. Robinson is Senior Anglican Chaplain and Lecturer in Theology at the University of Leeds. His interests are business and medical ethics, and pastoral theology. Other books include: *Serving Society - The Social Responsibility of Business; The Decision Makers - Ethics for Engineers; Agape, Moral Meaning and Pastoral Counselling; and Case Studies in Business Ethics.*

Acknowledgements

I would like to acknowledge the work of all who helped this book to come about. In particular I want to thank Richenda Milton-Thompson for her eagle eye, patience, good humour and great sense of order in the preparation of the manuscript. Ian Purvis, who is so knowledgeable on this subject, also made a number of very helpful suggestions.

Thanks too to the British Medical Association, and to the American Association for Retired Persons for permission to reproduce the material contained in Appendices I and II.

Preface

Kevin Kendrick died in September 2001 at the age of 40. He and I had just finished the first draft of this book. It is a mark of the man that he had four publishing projects unfinished. His creativity, enthusiasm and energy were such that he was always looking to the next project. Kevin could never have left this life in a tidy way, with everything complete, and doubtless he will be urging St Peter to consider what heavenly projects have not been covered.

Kevin's journey was ongoing, a remarkable example of lifelong learning. In amongst all the books, which marked him out as a rising expert in the fields of palliative care, care of the dying, and spirituality and healthcare, he was about to take on a PhD. Where would he have found the time? His head doubted there was any. His heart told him differently, and urged him on not only to develop his academic rigour, but also to maintain his high standard of professional practice and teaching, and to fulfil his love for his wife Pauline and two sons Steven and Paul. There is no doubt that his heart ruled. Sometimes this led to errors of judgement, such as his support for Liverpool Football Club. More often than not, though, it informed a rigorous decision making process, and critical reflection, enabling him to develop an academic life that did not simply embody standards and tradition but above all humanity. Because of this, Kevin's pastoral concern for his students was second to none.

Kevin was a big man, with a big heart and a creative mind, who fortunately for all who knew him never quite 'grew up'. I say fortunately because that gave us a man of grace and gentleness, of mischievous humour and charm, of utter realism and deep faith. It is precisely because of these qualities that he was able to reflect so effectively on dying and gaze, unblinking, into the face of death.

Simon J. Robinson
Leeds, 2001

Introduction

The practice of making living wills, or advance directives about treatment or refusal of treatment, has not become widespread in Great Britain. In contrast, the United States of America have embraced the idea and practice with enthusiasm, as embodying the individual's right to involvement in treatment at the end of life, in particular when he or she is no longer competent to make a contemporary decision about treatment. Hence that right is enshrined in both Federal and State law.

But what does it actually mean to have such a right? Does it make any real difference to the practice of care that is offered to individuals who are unable to make their own decisions about treatment? How do we balance the rights and autonomy of patients with the professional judgements of the medical profession, judgements which might be based on awareness of situation and possibilities unavailable to patients when their original directives were made? If the right is embedded in law what might the legal pitfalls be for the medical practitioner and how might awareness of these affect the care given? In all this, the rights of many different groups – patients, families, health care practitioners – begin to be articulated.

Doubts begin to creep in, and with those doubts, fears. At one level these are fears about how we might face the end of life, fears about loss of dignity, about the possible experience of suffering and pain, even though we may not be fully aware at the end. At another level there are the fears of not having one's voice heard. It is very hard for most of us to contemplate that end, and even harder to feel reassured that our particular end will be a good one, that we will be treated as we wished.

In this book we aim to explore just how individuals might begin to find a voice in this process of dying, and be able to feel assured that such a voice will be heard. This is particularly relevant as these individuals lie there, completely dependent on the care of others who are often under intense pressure.

The overall argument of the book is that finding such a voice cannot be seen simply as a matter of autonomy and legal rights. Finding a voice begins with the practice of telling our story, sharing our narrative, with our medical practitioner and with our relatives. And such a story is not simply a matter of deciding what treatment we wish to refuse. It is also about our values and underlying belief systems, how we view ourselves and the fact of our mortality. Such a voice is found in dialogue, not simply through a written statement. The written statement can be the focus of that dialogue, and the point of continuity, enabling all those involved in treatment, family and friends, to continue that dialogue, however brief it may be. We argue for living wills then, but not as expressing a legal right and not as something that can of itself solve all the problems surrounding ensuring a good death. Rather, we argue for living wills as a focus of dialogue and narrative.

In turn we hope that this will help to provide focus for families and medical practitioners, so that such reflections might become part of continuing medical dialogues. Ideally, this all becomes part of a learning cycle where family members are able to reflect openly at key times and build up an awareness of the needs and values of each other.

This was well summed up recently in the death of my father. My 17-year-old son, Jamie, and I were there with him as he lost the battle against pneumonia. Because he had shared in this experience, my son quite naturally began to ask how I would like my end to be. 'What do you want me to do when you are like that? I mean we can't wait till then to decide.' Up to that point I had not felt the need to think about my end. Now my son was thinking about it for me and enabling me to begin to articulate not just how I want to be treated then, but also about what form my good end will take – reception of Holy Communion, background music from Mahler's Third Symphony, someone reading from Wisden's description of Yorkshire's first win in the County Cricket Championship in 33 years, and so on. All of this was more of a fantasy than a bill of rights, and was emerging from the empathy and the humour implicit in the family relationship. The living will can assist this process of reflection, but is no substitute for it.

In the light of such reflections then any thoughts about the so called living will can only take place in the context of how we view death and how we approach decision making about death and dying. As we shall see this does not mean that living wills should be simply a matter for the elderly. They are, however, about death and dying, and how the process of dying might maintain the dignity and integrity of the patient when he or she is not competent to make a decision about treatment that might be followed. Hence, the early chapters of this book focus on death and dying.

The first chapter of this book looks at how we approach death as human beings and society. It begins to focus in, not so much on the nature and problems of preparing a living will, as upon how we respond to death individually and in community. This is the context of living wills. The second chapter looks at how a good death is communicated. This is contrasted with the medicalisation of death. Chapter Three then examines the legal framework of the living will. Although there is no intention of the British government to follow the American lead there are nonetheless important legal precedents and implications which have to be made clear for the patient, for the family, and for the medical practitioner. What legal rights there are will be clarified here. Chapter Four begins to reflect on the underlying ethical issues, including definition of personhood, and autonomy versus paternalism. It incorporates an argument for shared governance as distinct from individualistic autonomy. Hence, if any coherent idea of moral rights does emerge, it relates to the right to be heard.

Finally, in Chapter Five we summarise the practice and consider how living wills might most effectively be used in the context of developing medical and family relationships. Major guidelines from the British Medical Association and other bodies are included in the Appendices.

1 Death and Dying: past and present trends

'Death is another transformation through which we move, an adventure to surpass all adventures, an opening, an incredible moment of growth, a graduation'. (Albery, Elliot and Elliot 1993:12)

You may not echo the sentiments offered by Albery and colleagues. For you, thoughts of dying may be dreadful, hideous and frightening. One day, however, they will cease to be unwanted intruders and form the final threads of your 'lived experience'. As such, death is a part of life that deserves some prior thought.

The purpose of this chapter is to 'capture the mood' by looking at death in Western culture through a historical perspective up to and including the present. Rather than detailing distinct epochs, the chapter seeks to offer a sense of the past that captures those changing social and cultural narratives about death and dying which inform the present and will, consequently, shape the future.

We spend a lot of time making plans and get frustrated when, despite our best efforts, things go wrong. Have you ever set off early for an important appointment only to be thwarted and made late by roadworks? How many times have you made a careful shopping list and returned home to find you left a vital item off? What about Christmas? Weeks spent planning for every eventuality, then a great aunt you haven't seen for years turns up with a beautiful present and you have nothing for her! All this shows that despite careful planning, things still go wrong; nothing is certain – or so they say. But one event is certain to happen: you will die.

Living wills and advance directives are essentially documented 'plans'. They indicate an individual has thought about those details and features that would, ideally, form the defining elements, context and situation of mortality. Within these themes, there is an assertion of autonomy and the importance of individual choice. The essence and ethos of the living will translates an individual's wishes to a critical situation when it is no longer possible for that individual to articulate

1

their own 'best interests'. In this respect, the living will provides a 'live' testament of consent that informs the limits of what may and may not be done in terms of medical treatment. The core feature here is that the document seeks to guard against futile medical interventions that would compromise the individual's dignity and humanity when such means cannot be readily justified in terms of a successful curative end.

Beyond seeking to provide a means of self-advocacy about the nature of treatment in a critical health scenario, the living will also seeks to address something that precedes death; it is a celebration of life. Dying is the crowning of life, the leaving of what gave being, purpose and meaning. At the time of death, it may not be possible for a person to embrace these sentiments but the living will exists to enshrine those qualities that have defined a person's living and ensure these are not compromised, ignored or denigrated at the moment of dying.

In the USA and UK we are not used to seeing death in this way. So such language can be seen as prosaic and unrealistic. Yet beyond these features, there is a growing body of influence that argues for a cultural shift that more readily embraces a way of living that is geared towards personal reflection and preparation about the nature of dying and death. As Smith (2000) reflects in an Editorial in the *British Medical Journal*:

> 'Are you ready to die? If not, then you might begin some preparation. Every *BMJ* reader will die this century, and death is constantly beside us. Montaigne urged, "One should be ever booted and spurred and ready to depart." Yet that has not been the attitude of the past 50 years, and modern medicine may even have had the hubris to suggest implicitly, if not explicitly, that it could defeat death. If death is seen as a failure rather than as an important part of life then individuals are diverted from preparing for it and medicine does not give the attention it should to helping people die a good death.'

The thrust of Smith's thinking challenges modern European attitudes about dying and death; in doing so, it fires a creative shot across the bows of convention that has traditionally treated all things about human demise as taboo. In the following section we seek to find out why this may be so.

2

Social taboo

The seminal writings of Elisabeth Kubler-Ross maintain it is extremely difficult for the human psyche to accept death as an unavoidable part of life. For example, she states:

> 'In simple terms, in our conscious mind we can only be killed, it is inconceivable to die of a natural cause or of old age. Therefore, we associate it with a bad act, a frightening happening, something that in itself calls for retribution'. (Kubler-Ross 1969:2)

The sobering and stark realisation that one day we will be no more has been a powerful theme for creating and maintaining the social notion that death should be treated as a taboo subject. Part of the reason behind this can be explained with reference to the existential; putting this in its most simple form, death and dying are treated as taboo because they signal finality. Dying is the process leading towards non-being and death is its state. Since existentialism is essentially concerned with the state of being and existence then the opposite of such is, by definition, the nemesis of the existential. These elements are further reflected and captured by Koestenbaum, as follows:

> 'The genuine death of myself is best described as the annihilation of all being. It is the image of total nothingness – the absence of any image whatsoever – and its fully conscious anticipation is suffused with deep anxiety and uncontrollable nausea'. (Koestenbaum 1971:140)

In short, death is not a popular subject. If you want to test this out, try telling friends who are not health professionals that you are reading a book essentially concerned with death. You may well find such a revelation is unlikely to inspire passionate, or even interested, discussion. This wishing to avoid talk of death is poignantly supported by the following remarks from a doctor who tried to bring the subject up in public:

> 'We're in a restaurant … when I ask the person next to me whether they ever think about dying. "No yuck" is the response … however hard I try, no one's keen to chat about death in the funny intimate way they will about other aspects of their lives. Death

remains resoundingly taboo but still, as far as we know, a universal experience. And most people, myself included, aren't very happy about it.' (Dillner 1995:16)

This reluctance to openly talk about issues concerning death mirrors much of modern cultural entrenchment that sees issues of death and dying as taboo; it is a way of seeing human demise as essentially a 'bad' thing. Such thinking is graphically displayed in the following words from Rollo May:

'Death is obscene, unmentionable and pornographic ... death is a nasty mistake. Death is not to be talked of in front of the children, nor talked about at all if we can help it.' (May 1969:24)

Of course, being a health professional does not offer immunity from the emotional labour that is often a part of caring for a person unto death. Writing about the feelings of nurse colleagues following the death of a 36-year-old woman from multiple organ failure, Brash and colleagues (1995) reported the following themes:

1 Some nurses had found it extremely difficult to care for a young woman who had so much to live for. This had led to some nurses avoiding the patient altogether. Further conversations revealed that some nurses identified similarities between the patient's life and their own. This was painful and put forward as another reason for avoiding her.
2 Nurses expressed a collective fear of being unable to cope with questions that the patient may have raised about her impending death; this was another reason why nurses felt uncomfortable with anything other than superficial conversations.
3 Another source of anxiety was communicating with the patient's family about her death; as one member of the team put it 'What do you say to a husband and daughter when their closest friend is about to die?'

In a pivotal piece, Menzies (1970) explored the challenges that face nurses when they meet difficult scenarios such as dealing with people in acute grief. This research argued that delivering care to a person up to death and then for their relatives or friends gave nurses a strong sense of their own mortality. Menzies' work showed that nurses employ various defence mechanisms for evading close contact with dying persons and call upon these again later to avoid relatives. Similar findings have been mirrored in more recent works (Littlewood 1993, McNamara *et al.* 1995).

The way that modern society views death is informed and influenced by social mores, fears, rites and rituals from the past. During the rest of this chapter, we will ask some key questions about issues relating to the context and rituals of death and dying. This will help us consider such issues as: 'Has the way we deal with death changed over time?'

To start this exploration, we will examine briefly the historical dimensions of death and dying in British society.

Death in the past

The first time we see the body of a dead person, especially if we have been involved in caregiving, can be quite harrowing. This professional proximity to death is quite out of keeping with the experience of most members of society. In modern times, many individuals reach adulthood without seeing a dead person.

Unfortunately, we sometimes meet students whose first encounter with a corpse is traumatic. This is often due to circumstances beyond the control of the student or trained staff. For example, we recently talked with a nursing student who had arrived early for a shift and decided to chat with patient she got on well with. Only the previous evening, the student had been talking with the patient about television programmes. Nobody had seen the student arriving early or they would have warned her of the situation. The act of walking into the room to find the patient dead and in a shroud was really upsetting. It is easy to see why her first encounter with death was such a shock.

In the past, death was a much more obvious and open aspect of the community's every day life. In previous ages, death was intrinsically woven to the fabric of life, in such a way that families and friends seemed constantly touched, either directly or indirectly, by its presence. Seeing a dead body, therefore, was a fairly frequent occurrence.

'Death was much more commonplace – stalking society, ever ready to strike people of all age groups through killer diseases, especially in epidemics which could suddenly ravage entire communities. Infant deaths were a common experience and most families expected to lose some of their children. And as most deaths occurred at home, the process of dying and the presence of a corpse in the house were not unfamiliar events.' (Cox 1989:183)

Throughout the ages, being buried alive was a focus of the fear surrounding death. Up to the start of the last century, it was common to leave the body to putrefy (Kendrick 1990). This was a sure way of ensuring the person was dead and allowed death to be graphically seen as a poignant part of everyday life. Unfortunately, it also contributed greatly to the spread of disease and epidemics.

Imagine the scene in a London street during the great plagues that beset Europe during the middle ages. Not only was death commonplace, it was also extremely visual as bodies were thrown onto a wagon to the sound of 'bring out yer dead'. Human waste was thrown out of windows and filth was everywhere. The rich would smell scented posies to try and dull their senses to the stench of death and decay that was everywhere (Hale 1993).

In the eighteenth century, accounts of 'live sepulture' (being buried alive) were frequently reported in medical journals. This was further supported by exhumations that revealed the inside of coffin lids to have scratch marks and indentations – obvious signs that the poor person had tried desperately to reach the outside world.

This terror of being buried alive was reflected in much of Edgar Allan Poe's eighteenth century writing. His chosen genre, that of gothic horror, lends itself easily to such themes. After reading one of Poe's short stories, a Russian nobleman Karnice-Karnicke, patented a coffin with particular features. Central to the coffin's design was a mechanism that could be activated to ring bells and display flags on the surface. This had the sole purpose of bringing the attention of the outside world to the plight of the entombed individual.

All of this must be placed in a historical context. Epidemics of plague, cholera and smallpox frequently led to people collapsing and giving every appearance of being dead. It was not until 1874 that it became necessary to register deaths in Britain and even then the corpse did not have to be seen by a doctor. Given all this, it is easy to see why premature burial took place and why it was so feared by the living (*Encyclopaedia Britannica* 1992).

During previous centuries, as we have seen, death was a poignant and primal part of everyday life; it invariably took place in the home and affected all members of the family. During the next stage of this chapter, we will move into the twentieth century and look at seminal works that explore the way people and communities have dealt with death.

Death in the community

At the turn of the last century, the vast majority of deaths took place at home. There were reasons for this. Firstly, medical care was a luxury that most people could not afford. Men were sometimes covered by an employer's insurance, but this would not normally cover a wife and children.

Secondly, many hospitals had formerly been used as workhouses. From Elizabethan times, the workhouse was the last resort for paupers who were sick or destitute. Their aim was to provide shelter but at the same time to discourage people from relying on others. Hence, they were places of hard work and little relief. When the hospital had connotations of the workhouse then it certainly was not a place for illness let alone dying.

Criticism of the workhouse was a key theme in nineteenth century literature. In *A Christmas Carol*, the miserly Ebenezer Scrooge is asked by two men of business to give a small donation for the poor at Christmas. Scrooge asks if the workhouses are no longer open, to which one of the philanthropists replies: 'Many can't go there; and many would rather die' (Dickens 1846).

It is with memories of the workhouse that people lived and died at the beginning of the previous century.

Life and death in Staithes

In what has become a seminal study, Clark (1982) used a sociological analysis to explore the traditions and rituals surrounding death and dying in a small Yorkshire village, Staithes. Commenting upon the nature of death in this community, Clark stated:

'With the exception of accidental fatalities, death in Staithes in the early part of the century almost invariably took place in the home, where the sick and dying were the immediate responsibility of the family, to whom also befell the task of laying the dead to rest in an adequate and befitting manner.' (Cited in Dickenson and Johnson 1993:4)

Death in the early twentieth century

What is fascinating about this study is that everyone who knew the family seemed to have a role to play in the rites and rituals surrounding the funeral, burial and mourning:

1 After a person had died, the body was placed on something called the 'lying-out board'. This board was kept in the workplace of the local joiner who also performed the duties of undertaker.
2 The actual 'lying out' of the body was performed by experienced women of the village, recognised as being qualified to perform the task and who took great pride in their work.
3 The body was treated with great respect and reverence. After a thorough washing, the body was wrapped in a white sheet and put on the 'lying-out' board in the centre of the marital bed. The feet were covered with white woollen socks and a pillow placed on either side of the head. A sheet, folded into horizontal pleats, was placed over the whole body. Finally, a white handkerchief covered the face.
4 The period between the person dying and being buried was one of solemnity where all normal affairs where abandoned. Curtains were drawn across windows and mirrors covered over. Family members took turns, during the night, to sit with the body.
5 One woman, known as the 'bidder', would go throughout the village announcing the time and place of the funeral; this would involve knocking on every door in the village giving the pronouncement.

Meanwhile, other women would be busy making funerary foods. An example of this was something called 'funeral biscuits', a special sweet served with port on the day of the burial.

6 Following the funeral, family and friends met back at the house for a funeral tea. This was the time when mirrors and pictures were uncovered and the curtains partially opened.

7 After the funeral there were clear social sanctions placed upon the bereaved; these had to be carefully observed. This was a progressive passage from mourning to a gradual re-emergence into the full life of the community. For women, this was a particularly poignant period. In Staithes, women did not attend church for as much as a year. Indeed, appearance outside of the house was frowned upon and thought to be disrespectful.

More permanent reminders were kept of the person who had died. This would include the framing of large cards that contained biographical details of the deceased. Clark commented upon this particular aspect of mourning ritual:

> 'Grim reminders they must have been to a community where death was a frequent and untimely visitor.' (Cited in Dickenson and Johnson 1993:7)

Clark's work offers us some invaluable insights into the nature of dying, death, loss and mourning in the early years of the twentieth century.

Death in the late twentieth century

What is particularly interesting about Clark's work is that it also examines death and its various rites and rituals in the Staithes of his own day. Commenting upon the nature of death in contemporary Staithes, Clark states:

> 'Perhaps the most significant innovation is the emergence of a number of specialist organisations which increasingly concern themselves with the processes of death and dying. It is a transformation which has stripped the family of one of its traditional functions, so that some of the familial and communal rituals previously associated with the death of a villager have disappeared

beneath a general trend towards standardisation.' (Dickenson and Johnson 1993:8)

In essence, Clark's comments point towards modern death being a compartmentalised and commercial affair. The death may no longer occur at home, rather a person may die in the hospital or care home. Thus, the former ritual of 'lying-out' the body is performed by the nurse or funeral director and people pay their 'last respects' at the memorial house. There is no longer any place for the 'bidder' as the funeral director will place news of the death in the obituary column of the local newspaper. In modern Staithes, the funeral director will order the flowers and wreaths, even arrange with outside caterers to make the funeral tea.

Funeral directors play an invaluable role in shaping the rituals surrounding modern death. However, this form of death culture separates the bereaved from the practical aspects of preparing for the funeral. Important and intimate elements of collective mourning are lost forever.

All this has to be measured against other social trends. The changing shape of the family, different work patterns and the acceptance of consumerism all make the work of the funeral director seem convenient and necessary for the modern lifestyle. Indeed, while the community used to play a collective role in preparing for the funeral, the modern psyche might find such an idea distasteful, mainly because of its close association with death. A century ago, death was a proximal and unavoidable part of every day life, now we have the means to make it a much more hidden and clinical affair. Taking a slightly different approach, Walter (1990:33) argues that it is not that people find death difficult to face but that modern society seldom offers opportunities to confront it:

'Death is not very much present today. If the bereaved person finds others embarrassed, crossing to the other side of the street, I suspect it is not so much because they dare not, cannot confront death, but because they have had little practice at it, do not know what to do, are scared of saying the wrong thing.' (Walter 1990:33)

What we have seen is that death has become separate from the fabric of everyday human existence. Death still happens, thousands of people die every day in Britain, but most people do not see it in the 'raw' sense that was described by Clark in his study of Staithes.

Part of the popularity of television hospital documentaries is that they allow us to keep in touch with the essential theme that pain, suffering and death are part of life. In this way, we keep in touch with the subliminal notion that we will one day die. Whereas death was once constantly within the community, now we have individual opportunities to observe it in the privacy of our own homes through the television screen. Thus, that which was once shared by the community has become an isolated, private and slightly voyeuristic venture (Kendrick and Costello 2000).

What we have observed here is an important theme, death has shifted from being an experience shared by the whole community, to a much more insular and private affair. In the next part of this chapter, we will ask ourselves a question society continually hides from: 'What is it like to be dead?'

On being dead

Why do we find it so difficult to think of our own death? It is inevitable, unavoidable and absolute. Writing about the human fear of death, Hinton (1984) argues that it is healthy and has a biological basis. Taking this further, if we did not fear death then we would continually take risks that may be fatal, for life would hold neither individual or universal value. Thus, to ask such a blunt question as, 'What is it like to be dead?' certainly shuns established convention. Moreover, we can only surmise what death is like – nobody can detail the experience first hand.

The playwright, Tom Stoppard, has asked the question, 'What is it like to be dead?' In his acclaimed *Rosencrantz and Guilderstern are Dead*, he offers us this amusing and poignant insight:

'Do you ever actually think of yourself as actually dead, lying in a box with a lid on it? ... It's silly to be depressed by it. I mean one thinks of it like being alive in a box, one keeps forgetting to take into account the fact that one is dead …. which should make a difference …. shouldn't it? I mean, you'd never know how you were in a box, would you? It would be just like being asleep in a box. Not that I'd like to sleep in a box, mind you, not without any air – you'd wake up dead, for a start, and then where would you be? Apart from inside a box …. because you'd be helpless, wouldn't you? Stuffed in a box like that, I mean you'd be in there forever. Even taking into account the fact that you're dead, really …. I wouldn't think about it if I were you. You'd only get depressed. (*Pause*) Eternity is a terrible thought. I mean, where's it going to end?' (Stoppard 1967:62)

This graphic piece of writing starts of by asking us not to be depressed by the thought of being dead, of lying in the box. Then there is a shift in emphasis as the reality of existence in a coffin begins to dawn, indeed, the sheer futility of the idea starts to become obvious. Even if it were possible, the notion of spending eternity in a coffin starts to fill the speaker with dread. There are images here that fit in with our earlier discussion of premature burial.

Stoppard's writing is so illustrative and dynamic because it penetrates established social taboos. Asking questions about the experience of being dead rips at the fabric of established convention. Such writing is challenging because it subliminally engages the reader or listener to confront their own primal fears and beliefs about death.

Eternal youth and life

All of this must be placed in a modern context where youth and beauty are the gods of the market place. In an age when plastic surgery, beauty and fitness industries cater for a multi-billion pound market the subliminal message is clear: 'We want to live forever.' Such themes can only reinforce the notion that death is, in some perverse manner, a failure.

Exploring notions like this is vital to our work as health professionals. If cultural norms dictate that youth and beauty are desirable and can be purchased through the lotion, potion, gym or surgeon's knife, what kind of arena can we hope to create for the dying?

In the USA and much of modern Europe the panacea for eternal youth and life is a definite objective. In recent times, attempts to beat death have taken dramatic turns. There are now people paying substantial sums of money to have their bodies frozen in extreme temperatures after their death – this is known as cryogenics. The chief purpose for this is to preserve the body until a cure for the disease has been found. It is then hoped the body can be defrosted, treated and the person restored to health and vitality.

Other people are investing heavily in more traditional scientific methods. Writing in *The Sunday Times*, Tim Kelsey says of an 81-year-old American, Miller Quarles:

'Quarles has committed himself to a Faustian quest to buy more life. He has invested much of his fortune in a revolutionary research project that may have just identified the biological clock that determines when we die. The work has been hailed as one of the most important discoveries in modern science.' (Kelsey 1996:1)

Such developments can only fuel the notion that death is wrong, unacceptable and, ultimately, a failure. What is so poignant here is a message that death is in some way unnatural. Yet, as we have already explored, death is as much a part of life as birth. They are just different sides of the same coin. This is an image so important to the ethos underpinning the care we give to dying individuals and their loved ones.

Concluding reflections

The whole thrust of this chapter has been to explore human reactions and attitudes towards death. In doing this, we have covered a number of themes that relate to the fears, rituals and rites that have enshrined the management of death. What has emerged is that contemporary society no longer has a close proximity to death. With this the idea of collective mourning, where the whole community played a part in the customs of death, has disappeared forever. This cultural shift has made death distant and foreign to everyday life.

We have also seen that developments like cryogenics create a cultural image where death is to be shunned and seen, subliminally, as a failure. Yet death is a natural process. If we begin to see it as a failure, what will this mean for the care we give to dying patients? Death is not a failure, it is the final event of life.

References

Albery, N., Elliot, G., Elliot, J. (1993) *The Natural Death Handbook.* Virgin Publishing, London.

Brash, J., McKenna, C., Kendrick, K. (1995) 'Freedom to grieve: a nursing response.' In Kendrick, K.D., Weir, P., Rosser E. (eds) *Innovations in Nursing Practice.* Edward Arnold, London.

Clark, D. (1982) *Between Pew and Pulpit.* Cambridge University Press, Cambridge.

Cox, C. (1989) *Sociology: an introduction for nurses, midwives and health visitors.* Butterworth Heinemann, London.

Dickens, C. (1846) *A Christmas Carol.* Reissued 1994 by The Folio Society, London.

Dickenson, D., Johnson, M. (1993) *Death, Dying and Bereavement.* Sage Publications, London, in association with The Open University, Milton Keynes.

Dillner, L. (1995) 'No death please we're British.' *The Guardian,* 9 September: 16.

Encyclopaedia Britannica (1992) *Encyclopaedia Britannica.* University of Chicago, Encyclopaedia Britannica Inc, Chicago.

Hale, J. (1993) *The Civilisation of Europe in the Renaissance.* Harper Collins, London.

Hinton, J. (1984) *Dying.* Penguin, Harmondsworth.

Kelsey, T. (1996) 'Who wants to live forever?' *The Sunday Times* (News Review), 7 January: 1.

Kendrick, K., Costello, J. (2000) 'Healthy viewing? Experiencing life and death through a voyeuristic gaze.' *Nursing Ethics*, 7 (1): 15–22.

Kendrick, K. (1990) *Partners in Passing: ethical aspects of nursing the dying person*. Unpublished MSc Dissertation, University of Liverpool.

Koestenbaum, P. (1971) *The Vitality of Death: essays in existential psychology and philosophy*. Westport, Greenwood.

Kubler-Ross, E. (1969) *On Death and Dying*. Tavistock Publications, London.

Littlewood, J. (1993) 'The denial of death and rites of passage in contemporary societies.' In Clark, D. (ed) *The Sociology of Death*. Blackwell, Oxford.

May, R. (1969) *Love and Will*. Dell, New York.

McNamara, B., Waddell, C., Colvin, M. (1995) 'Threats to the good death: the cultural context of stress and coping among hospice nurses.' *Sociology of Health and Illness*, 17: 224–244.

Menzies, N. (1970) *Communication and Stress: a nursing perspective*. Macmillan, London.

Smith, R. (2000) 'A good death.' *British Medical Journal*, 320: 129–130.

Stoppard, T. (1969) *Rosencrantz and Guildenstern are Dead*. Faber & Faber, London.

Walter, T. (1990) *Funerals and How to Improve Them*. Hodder and Stoughton, London.

2 A Good Death

'We believe it is time to break the taboo and to take back control of an area [death] which has been medicalised, professionalised, and sanitised to such an extent that it is now alien to most people's daily lives' (Age Concern 1999:41).

'Good death': defining features

One of the key themes in the previous chapter was that most people no longer experience the communal immediacy of dying and death that was familiar to former generations (Field 1996). Such themes are reflected in the sobering thought that two-thirds of Britons now die in hospital (Walter 1994). Some commentators talk as if this 'medicalisation' of death was a recent phenomenon concerned with technological developments, for example:

> 'This "Displacement of the site of death" from the home to the hospital has occurred without any planning or intending it. This societal trend has occurred not by design but rather because of the irresistible movement of technological development.' (Krakauer 1996:22; see also Clark 2002)

Placing the medicalisation of death firmly within a twentieth century context is out of kilter with the historical schema. As Porter (1989) has pointed out, people have been concerned with medicine's controlling influence of and relationship with death for hundreds of years. In supporting his position, Porter quotes Thomas Sheridan's writing from the 1760s:

> 'Very few people now die. Physicians take care to conceal people's danger from them. So they are carried off, properly speaking, without dying; that is to say, without being sensible of it.' (Porter 1989:89)

All of this signifies a truism – life's unavoidable aspect is that death calls inclusively upon all who enjoy the human condition. Given the inevitability of mortality, it is important to engage critically with those features that lend themselves towards the definition of a 'good death'.

Such thinking seems immediately questionable since how can death ever be 'good'? Since time immemorial, philosophers and theologians have given equal attention to two juxtaposed questions: is death a bad thing? And, what is a good death? (Levi 1998). Perhaps the choice of such a value-laden word as 'good' is appropriate in the context of death since its certainty suggests that to seek anything other than a 'good' death seems, at the very least, unfortunate (one certainly would not rush to secure a 'bad' death). As health professionals, it would certainly be our wish that patients have a 'good' death and that we seek to attend to this end through the provision of our professional acumen and focus. Of course, there are some deaths that will always be unavoidably and twistingly dreadful. Nothing will ever lessen, for example, the devastating impact surrounding death from an unsuspected ruptured aortic aneurysm or a lymphoma that suddenly haemorrhages while attached to a vital vessel. The defining features of a 'bad' death are readily identifiable and frightening: uncontrollable pain, loss of control, lack of choice, loss of dignity and no opportunity to say 'goodbye' to loved ones (hence the horror associated with grieving a sudden death). Given these elements, there is little surprise to find that opposite features have been identified by The Age Concern report *The Future of Health and Care of Older People* (1999) as being the core themes that constitute a 'good' death (see Box 2.1).

Box 2.1 *Principles of a good death*

- To know when death is coming, and to understand what can be expected
- To be able to retain control of what happens
- To be afforded dignity and privacy
- To have control over pain relief and other symptom control

- To have choice and control over where death occurs (at home or elsewhere)

- To have access to information and expertise of whatever kind is necessary

- To have access to any spiritual or emotional support required

- To have access to hospice care in any location, not only in hospital

- To have control over who is present and who shares the end

- To be able to issue advance directives which ensure wishes are respected

- To have time to say goodbye, and control over other aspects of timing

- To be able to leave when it is time to go, and not to have life prolonged pointlessly

(Age Concern 1999:42)

Underlying these principles are some key concepts:

- **Control.** Patients should be able to direct their own ending in some way whether they are aware or not.
- **Freedom.** The patient at some point in the process should have been able take an informed decision about treatment. This is not simply freedom to choose but freedom to decide in relation to their physical and social environment.
- **Respect.** This can be defined as respect for the patient as subject – autonomous decision maker.
- **Care.** This involves care for the whole person, requiring both good symptom control and attention to the person's meaning system, both values and beliefs. It also involves a chronological awareness of the person, taking account of their past life and present situation. Significantly, the living will or advance directive gives attention to this dimension of the patient.

Most of the elements offered as constituents of a 'good' death are contingent upon honest communication between the dying person and all those individuals, lay and professional, involved with the delivery of care. For example, a 'living will' has little hope of representing the 'best interests' of the dying person if its existence has not been communicated to all relevant parties. Such good communication is central to palliative care, necessary from the moment of breaking bad news to collaboration with families, until the final moments of treatment or withdrawal of treatment.

Communication

It's good to talk – but better to listen

Communication is vital for human flourishing; without it people would find themselves in a social vacuum devoid of essence or meaning. Communication is, therefore, essential to the formation and development of social reality. As health professionals, communication forms the heart of our dealings with patients. Imagine how sterile, passive and empty words such as 'enable', 'empower' and 'support' would be if communication could not translate them to workable themes in the relationships we share with patients. The relevance of these sentiments is reflected in the following statement:

> 'The most important single factor in the delivery of health care is the competence of the people to deliver it and their ability to communicate.' (Hall 1984:129)

Anything that causes a threat to an individual's life and future can result in the person being cast into the throes of uncertainty and fear. In health care delivery, practitioners are often faced with the daunting task of giving information that confronts an individual's most fundamental and essential fears about illness, death, dying and the unknown. Sometimes this process is described by the term 'breaking bad news' (Buckman 1993).

Defining 'bad news'

The term 'bad news' is used in everyday language to describe a whole range of negative events. Even in health care settings, the interpretation

19

of what constitutes 'bad news' is largely subjective and dependent upon patients' individual perceptions; for example, some people are untroubled by being told they need an injection, whereas others see it as very 'bad news'. However, in more specific terms, Rob Buckman argues that breaking bad news usually involves giving traumatic information that has a major and often irreversible impact upon a patient's life:

> 'By "bad news" I mean any information likely to alter drastically a patient's view of his or her future (whether at the time of diagnosis or when facing the failure of curative intention). Naturally, how bad the news is will depend to some extent on the patients' expectations at the time, on how ill they actually feel, and on whether or not they already know or suspect their diagnosis or current state.' (Buckman 1993:23)

There is a vast range of possible scenarios and settings in which bad news is given. Three key areas that frequently cause practitioners anxiety when dealing with this difficult and sensitive issue are:

- When a patient asks the question, 'Have I got cancer?'
- Dealing with collusion (for example, when relatives or friends demand that the news of a poor prognosis is kept from the patient).
- Breaking news of a patient's sudden death to their relative or friend over the phone.

'Have I got cancer?'

The consequences of not being truthful when a person asks this question can be catastrophic. Sometimes practitioners enter into the fragile world of word games to try and avoid a direct confrontation with the truth. Many vague and evasive responses are given to the question, 'Have I got cancer?' (Kendrick and Weir 1996:95). For example:

- 'I thought the doctor told you that it was a tumour – I never heard the word cancer mentioned'
- 'What sort of a question is that to ask when you are looking so well?'

Such responses are deceitful and threaten the foundations of the therapeutic relationship. A person who has the courage to ask so plainly about their illness deserves to be answered in a similar fashion. This does not mean that revealing the truth to a person about cancer will be easy – either for the patient or the nurse, but it does free the individual to face the situation with an open and informed gaze. Such an approach is supported by Hebblethwaite (1991) who argues, 'There is a recognition that "the truth" will almost inevitably be painful and almost nothing can make it painless, but we must be careful not to underestimate anyone's inner resources'.

Sometimes patients do not ask such a direct question as 'Have I got cancer?' Rather, they may ask vague questions that need further exploration and clarification before an answer is given. Writing about the way in which bad news should be gently and slowly revealed to patients, Maguire and Faulkner (1993) offer the following insights:

> 'It is important to accept that you cannot soften the impact of bad news since it is still bad news however it is broken. The key to breaking it is to try to slow down the speed of the transition from a patient's perception of himself as being well to a realisation that he or she has a life-threatening disease'. (Maguire and Faulkner 1993:180)

Box 2.2 shows, in dialogue form, how such themes can be applied in a practice setting.

Box 2.2 *Communicating bad news: dialogue in practice*

Nurse: I'm afraid it's more than just an ulcer …

Patient: What do you mean more than just an ulcer?

Nurse: Some of the cells are abnormal

Patient: Abnormal?

Nurse: The cells look cancerous under the microscope

Patient: You mean I've got cancer?

Nurse: I am afraid so, yes.

(Adapted from Maguire and Faulkner 1993)

Applying such themes in the practice setting can help deliver bad news in a humane and focused way. Such demands place a heavy weight upon the art of communication and celebrate the importance of listening and non-verbal communication in the breaking of 'bad news'.

The importance of listening and body language

Listening is a vital part of the process of communication when caring for people who are dying. In the end, it is not just what we say to people, it is how we listen to them. Listening involves a range of qualities and activities. First, it requires that we see the other person as *important*. We are prepared to give this other person our time. Second, it requires that we are *interested* in the other person. We cannot listen if we are bored by what we hear. Third, we must be prepared to *work* at listening. Most of us are not born good listeners. We have to put in the effort to become better. Fourth, we must be able to separate the problems of other people from our own problems. What another person tells us about him or herself does not necessarily relate to us. We do not have to assume that what people tell us *affects* us. We must learn, perhaps, to distinguish between another person's problems and our own. If we do not do this, we will find that we confuse ourselves and we fail to listen carefully. Listening, then, is a curious combination of giving our complete attention to another person and also of being able to detach ourselves a little from the other person (Burnard and Kendrick 1998).

To listen to another person is the most human of actions. In health care it is a crucial skill. Listening refers to the process of hearing what the patient is saying. Hearing encompasses not only the words that are being used but also the non-verbal aspects of the encounter. Adding one further element to this, the term 'attending' refers to the practitioner's skill in paying attention to the patient.

Hargie, Saunders and Dickson (1994) list the general functions of listening in the following way:

- To focus specifically upon the messages being communicated by the other person
- To gain full, accurate understanding of the other person's communication

- To convey interest, concern and attention
- To encourage full, open and honest expression.

Gerard Egan (1982) offered an acronym for recalling the important aspects of non-verbal activity during the listening process. Egan suggested that, in Western countries, these behaviours are associated with effective listening. The acronym that Egan offers is as follows:

S: Sit *squarely* in relation to the client
O: Maintain an *open* position
L: *Lean* slightly forward
E: Maintain comfortable *eye contact* with the client
R: *Relax* while listening.

Sitting squarely means sitting opposite the person who is being listened too, rather than next to them. In this way, the one doing the listening can see *all* of the other person and can observe the non-verbal behaviours of the talker. The position also demonstrates interest in the other person.

An open position means that the listener does not have their arms crossed. Such behaviour can create real barriers to effective communication because 'closed' physical positioning can often be construed as being defensive.

Eye contact should be steady and appropriate. No one wants to be stared at but neither do they want to feel that the person who is supposed to be listening to them will look anywhere but at them. Eye contact may also depend upon the relative status of the pair involved. Finally, the listener should try to sit quietly and be relaxed. When listening to another person, we do not have to be constantly rehearsing what we will say next. Nor do we have to relate everything that is said to us and to our own thoughts and feelings.

Egan's guidelines on how to sit when listening to another person may be useful as a baseline. Clearly, no one wants to talk to a person who sits and looks like a statue. On the other hand, it does not help very much to sit, lounge and fidget when listening. The SOLER acronym serves as a gentle reminder and guide on how to listen effectively.

There is a danger, if these sorts of behaviours are adhered to too literally, that the patient will *notice* the 'forced' behaviour of the practitioner. These sorts of behaviours are useful if they become 'natural' to the user but less so if the user feels uncomfortable with them.

Box 2.3 *The skills of effective listening*

Hargie *et al.* (1994) offer the following basic guidelines to be borne in mind when listening:

- Get physically prepared to listen ...

- Be mentally prepared to listen objectively ...

- Use spare thought time positively ...

- Avoid interrupting the speaker where possible ...

- Organise the speaker's messages into appropriate categories and, where possible, into chronological order ...

- Remember that listening is hard work.

Effective listening

It is a fact that we have to work at listening. However, Woolf and colleagues (1983) offer the following points to try and facilitate effective listening. Their ten points are as follows:

- Do not stereotype the speaker
- Avoid distractions
- Arrange a conducive environment (adequate ventilation, lighting, seating etc.)
- Be psychologically prepared to listen
- Keep an open, analytical mind, searching for the central thrust of the speaker's message
- Identify supporting arguments and facts
- Do not dwell on one or two aspects at the expense of others
- Delay judgment or refutation, until you have heard the entire message
- Don't formulate your next question while the speaker is relating information
- Be objective.

Listening, then, is the act of forgetting one's self and giving full and caring attention to another person (Burnard and Kendrick 1998). It involves a non-judgemental quality and an ability to be 'free floating' in one's attention to the other person. For here is a paradox: if we listen *too* closely to *everything* that another person says, we are likely to lose the 'drift' of what they are saying. We need to keep a *general* attention to the totality of what they are saying, while keeping an eye out for the important details.

If communication between health professionals, dying people and their loved ones is less than open and honest, then it threatens the therapeutic relationship. If veracity is compromised trust becomes the casualty. This is seen most vividly in the moral quagmire that is called 'collusion'.

Communication and the ethical problem of collusion

It may be said, with reasonable certainty, that truth and honesty form central themes in relationships between patients and practitioners. In most cases, to deal in anything other than the truth can violate trust and destroy any hope of a therapeutic association. These themes find particular resonance in the light of the following case study.

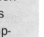

Case Study 2.1 Jamie

Jamie is 15 years old and has been suffering with early morning nausea and vomiting, violent headaches and an inability to concentrate on his work at school. The general practitioner thought this was a virus that would pass in a week or two. However, the symptoms progressively got worse and included faints and a feeling of numbness down the left side of his body. Jamie was immediately referred to the regional neurological centre for investigations.

The result of these investigations is devastating. Jamie has been found to have a particularly aggressive, malignant tumour. Unfortunately, the growth is fixed to vital structures, meaning surgery is not a viable option. Jamie's parents, Joanna and Michael, are extremely upset by this news. The consultant neurologist is gently honest, saying the most that can be done is to make Jamie as comfortable as possible in the time left to him. Joanna and Michael are enraged. Why can nothing be done for their son? 'There must be something you can do – he's only 15'. The dreadful reality is that nothing can be offered to Jamie and his parents except the fervent hope and desire that palliative care might keep him pain free and comfortable.

Five days after hearing the news of Jamie's prognosis, Joanna and Michael ask to see the senior sister, Pam. Looking drawn and exhausted, Joanna starts to plead with Pam. 'Sister, Mike and I have had a chance to think things through about Jamie. It's really nice that you feel able to say his illness will be closely watched and everything done to make him comfortable – that reassures us, but something else is really bothering us.'

Joanna starts to cry and Pam sits quietly waiting for her to carry on in her own time. Mike interjects, 'The point is that we don't want Jamie to know about his illness. At the moment he still thinks that he has a virus, he really couldn't take the news that there was nothing more which could be done ... so if he asks what is wrong he mustn't be told the truth, he just could not take it, for goodness sake, he's just a little boy'.

Joanna and Mike cling to each other, both weeping bitterly. Pam leaves them at what she felt was an intensely private moment. Outside the office, Pam ponders the dilemma which the team now face – do they really have the right to tell a 15-year-old boy that he is going to die when the people who love and know him better than anybody else plead against it? Do health professionals have a moral mandate to override such knowledge?

Box 2.4 *Collusion – defining features*

- In health care, collusion usually involves a covert understanding between practitioners and relatives that the news of a poor prognosis is kept from a patient

- The conventions that inform normal interaction between people would not tolerate this form of behaviour

- However, such views are confronted when relatives or friends put forward powerful sentiments such as those seen in the previous case study

- Do health professionals have a moral mandate to override the wishes of relatives who know the patient more than we could ever hope to?

Relatives who seek collusion often argue that they are in a much better position to understand what their loved one can and cannot take. Reflecting upon the reasons why relatives put forward requests such that the truth of a poor prognosis be kept from the patient, Kendrick and Shea comment:

'A prognosis which indicates that death is inevitable confronts the most primal elements of the human condition. It is understandable that relatives sometimes request or even demand that such devastatingly "bad news" be kept from a loved one. The essential reason for this is to try and protect the dying person from the ravages inherent to such an announcement. Underpinning this is a firm belief that it is in the dying person's "best interests" not to know that death is approaching.' (Kendrick and Shea 1995:9)

What emerges from this is a convincing mandate from Jamie's parents to keep the truth from him. Initially this can take both a direct and indirect form. If Jamie were to ask specifically what was wrong with him then the health professional could omit to tell the truth by, for example, conveniently 'side stepping' the issue – a common ruse being 'I'll get the doctor to have a word with you'. Alternatively, the nurse may choose to take the more direct route and lie to Jamie by saying, for example, 'these viruses can take an eternity to clear up'. Approaches of this nature are usually offered under the guise of wanting to protect the patient from the truth. Despite the good intent that may support such themes, a host of ethical indicators highlight the harm that can emerge from such reasoning.

Truth

The dismissal of truth

The very nature of collusion means that truth will be a casualty. If practitioners and relatives enter into a covert understanding which alienates a dying person from knowledge of the prognosis then the threads of a therapeutic bond become violated. What can emerge from this is a scenario born of deceit and disingenuous encounters. The intent underpinning collusion is often to protect the dying person from the news of an inevitable death from an illness that cannot be cured. Unfortunately, once such a position is taken it can have dire repercussions for the dynamics between all those involved with the dying person. Reflecting these themes, Kendrick and Kinsella (1994) state, 'Once we have entered into the dangerous scenario of collusion it leads to a constant striving to avoid tumbling down the slippery slope into a swirling vortex of lies, misrepresentation and fabrication'.

Returning once more to the earlier scenario, Joanna and Mike would love to protect Jamie from the news of the brain tumour and what it will inevitably mean. However, the loss of autonomy and trust which can result from collusion can hardly be justified. The opportunity for Jamie to reflect on his life and make sense of it should not be robbed from him under the guise of beneficence. What this establishes is, that in colluding against the truth, relatives and practitioners deny the dying person the status of being a valued subject. In logical sequence, this inevitably means that the patient becomes an object. This shift in perception and emphasis has a long history in the way that dying people are treated (Hanson 1994). The cliché that is often used to highlight this shift from valued subject to object is when a practitioner refers to the patient as, for example, 'the CA in the side ward'.

There are usually two main reasons that are put forward to support collusion:

- Adherence to the principle 'do no harm'
- Patients do not want to know the truth.

The notion that health care delivery can ever be 'free of harm' is Utopian. A person who has the courage to ask plainly about their mortality deserves an honest answer. This does not mean that revealing the truth to a person about impending death will be easy – either for the patient or for the nurse – but it does free the dying person to face death with an open and informed gaze.

In relation to the second premise in defence of collusion, there is little doubt that some patients do not want to be told the truth about their impending mortality. However, Bok (1978) revealed that 80 per cent of patients wanted to know the truth about their condition and prognosis. Supporting this approach, Gillon (1986:105) states, 'There are difficulties to overcome, but avoiding deceit is a basic moral norm, defensible from several moral perspectives'. Similar themes are echoed by Faulder (1985:89) who argues 'In asking patients to trust them it would seem only fair that doctors should reward that trust by dealing honestly with them'. All of this must be tempered by the notion that news of a poor diagnosis should always be revealed as gently as possible. This should be in a manner dictated by the patient, however strongly their well-meaning relatives wish to protect them from the truth about their approaching death.

If we do decide to collude with relatives and keep the truth of impending death from a patient, this can violate any of the therapeutic themes that have been established. The only substantive reason that would justify a dying person being left in a state of unknowing is a clear expression of not wanting to hear about a terminal prognosis.

The importance of truthful dialogue

A key task of this chapter has been to examine the main moral issues that emerge from the issue of collusion. We have seen that the practical considerations that emerge from this question cannot simply be viewed as a matter of doing good and avoiding harm. In relation to truth telling, revealing to patients that their death is fast approaching may evoke feelings of horror and disbelief among relatives who sought collusion. However, there may also be a feeling of relief that at least something has been found which can be labelled and seen as the cause of illness. Professional experience often reveals that patients find the 'not knowing' more unbearable than the harsh reality that life is coming to an end (Hanson 1994). Being honest about a prognosis that reveals life will end does give the patient a tremendous blow. However, such news, if offered gently and with a velvet glove, is easier to take than the devastation of trust and honesty which lying, deceit and collusion would mean for the dying person.

Therapeutic means to a 'good' death

The nature and manner of dying has consistently been a reported source of fear and concern among patients (Klagsburn 1981, Scott 1995). To offer a therapeutic presence at such times to dying people demands a core, defining focus. Perhaps this hub of caring is poignantly reflected in the following definition:

> 'Palliative care is defined as comprehensive, interdisciplinary care of patients and families facing a terminal illness, focusing primarily on comfort and support. Key aspects include meticulous symptom control; psychosocial and spiritual care; a personalised management plan that maximises patient-determined quality of life; family oriented care that extends through the time of bereavement; and delivery of coordinated services, especially in the home but also in hospital, extended care facilities, day care centres, and specialised units'. (Billings 2000:555)

Our task as health professionals is to give these themes definition within our professional context and situation. In essence, this embraces a holistic approach whereby the practitioner seeks to empathise with the 'lived experience' of the dying person and their family. This further translates itself to the caring milieu through helping the patient and family adjust to changes in lifestyle caused by the transition into palliative care, onto and including the dying process, followed by appropriate bereavement care thereafter (Karrer 1996).

Palliative care

Beyond these themes, recent times have also witnessed advances across the broad remit of palliative care. These developments have offered commensurate opportunities for practitioners, especially nurses, to advance their practice, building and extending beyond the scope of those defining features mentioned so far within a multidisciplinary framework (Hearn and Higginson 1998). This is particularly so in relation to pain management.

Multidisciplinary and complementary approaches to symptom control and pain management

Recent changes in the law relating to the prescription of medicines will mean increasingly that nurses will have an advanced role to play in the management of pain (Foley 1999) and symptom control when caring for people during the palliative process (Bagnall 1996, Ryecroft-Malone *et al.* 2000). Nearly all of the pain experienced by people suffering a terminal illness can be adequately relieved by simple, easily understood routines of medication in tablet from which are likely to have few or no troublesome side effects (Abrahm 1999). However, clinical practice continues to be characterised by unrelieved pain, illogical prescribing of pain-relieving drugs, and widespread fear of the side effects of strong opioid drugs to relieve pain. Billings (2000) has called this anxiety about opioid use 'opiophobia' and suggests the following may complement the traditional use of opioids:

- The use of bisphosphonate tablets to prevent and treat secondary tumours in the bone and associated pain in a variety of cancers
- New opioid preparations, particularly long-acting forms to be given as tablets or by injection, that simplify drug administration and may have other advantages
- Systemically administered local anaesthetics (either applied to the skin or taken in tablet form). These may include parenteral lignocaine (lidocaine) or oral mexiletine, and ketamine for neuropathic pain
- Psychostimulant drugs to counteract the sedative effect of opioids
- Topical local anaesthetic creams, such as Emla cream (lignocaine and prilocaine), to reduce skin pain from medical procedures
- Radiotherapy.

Beyond these elements, palliative care also affords the opportunity to address pain through methods that can act as adjuncts to traditional pharmacological means. In this respect, complementary therapies offer a broad range of interventions that can help a dying person in relation to pain and symptom control (Penson 1991, Kendrick 1999). The following identifies just some of the complementary therapies that emerge from the literature:

- Abdominal massage in the treatment of constipation when there is no indication of intestinal obstruction (Emly 1993)
- Therapeutic touch for physical, emotional and spiritual pain (Glasson 1996)
- Aromatherapy for agitation and anxiety (Gilliland 1999)
- Reflexology: a research paper by Hodgson (2000:35) reported the following impact of reflexology upon patients with advanced cancer: 'The areas which demonstrated the greatest improvement were appetite, breathing, constipation, diarrhoea, fears of the future, pain, nausea, sleep, communication and tiredness'.

Communication and care

What we have noted in this chapter is that the features of a good death are, to some extent, reliant upon people being able to make informed choices. The way in which health professionals can facilitate this is almost entirely through communication. Communication that is open, cogent and focused will go a long way towards preventing the occurrence of those ethical dilemmas we have visited concerning the breaking of 'bad news' and its all too frequent corollary of collusion. The Age Concern report on the future of health care reinforces this conclusion and recommends that the underlying values of palliative care are 'widely shared and adhered to' in medical and nursing education and amongst all who care for older people (Age Concern 1999:43).

Age Concern also note the importance of developing 'death education' in a much broader way. At one level this might involve encouraging the good practice of, for instance, the Natural Death Centre. The Centre has developed a 'death plan' proforma that enables recording of the person's wishes about treatment in the event of terminal illness, who should be present at the end, and how the end might be managed, even down to the music that might be played (Smith 2000). Such developments all contribute to the exercise of informed choice, and increased confidence that the wishes of the patient will be respected. In turn they enable reflection on and articulation of wishes and central values.

In addition the Age Concern report recommends that 'death education' be extended to schools. Education in citizenship, sexual relationships and moral decision making are an accepted part of the responsibility of schools. This could easily be extended to include ' positive consideration of ageing, and understanding the nature of dying and the rituals of death' (Age Concern 1999:45).

Of course none of this is simply learning about the nature of death and how to respond to dying, grieving and mourning. More fundamentally it is about developing the capacity to respond to the needs and wishes of the living about an experience which is inescapably part of what it means to be human, and increasing our awareness of how such meaning might be embodied. A vital part of this communication is the so called living will and we now turn to consider how interest in it began, its legal status and how its practice might be developed.

References

Age Concern (1999) *The Future of Health and Care of Older People.* Age Concern, England, London.

Abrahm, J.L. (1999) 'Management of pain and spinal cord compression in patients with advanced cancer.' (For the ACP-ASIM End-of-life Care Consensus Panel) *Annals of Internal Medicine*, 13: 37–46.

Bagnall, P. (1996) 'Don't overlook the real progress on nurse prescribing.' *Nursing Standard*, 10 (20): 10.

Billings, J.A. (2000) 'Palliative care.' *British Medical Journal*, 321(7260): 555–558.

Bok, S. (1978) *Lying: moral choice in public and private lives.* Harvester Press, Brighton.

Buckman, R. (1993) 'Breaking bad news: why is it still so difficult?' In Dickenson, D., Johnson, M. (1993) *Death, Dying and Bereavement.* Sage Publications, London, in association with The Open University, Milton Keynes.

Burnard, P., Kendrick, K. (1998) *Ethical Counselling.* Arnold, London.

Clark, D. (2002) 'Between hope and acceptance: the medicalisation of dying.' *British Medical Journal,* 324 (13 April): 905–907.

Egan, G. (1982) *Exercises in Helping Skills.* Brookes/Cole, Monterey, CA.

Emly, M. (1993) 'Abdominal massage.' *Nursing Times,* 89(3): 34–36.

Faulder, C. (1985) *Whose Body is It? The troubling issue of informed consent.* Virago Press, London.

Field, D. (1996) 'Awareness and modern dying'. *Mortality,* 1(3): 255–266.

Foley, K.M. (1999) 'Advances in cancer pain.' *Archives of Neurology,* 56: 413–417.

Gillon, R. (1986) *Philosophical Medical Ethics.* John Wiley, Chichester.

Gilliland, I. (1999) 'Case report. Using aromatherapy as a therapeutic nursing intervention.' *Journal of Hospice and Palliative Nursing,* 1(4): 157–158.

Glasson, M. (1996) 'Therapeutic touch in palliative care.' *Canadian Nurse,* 92(1): 19.

Hall, J. (1994) *Psychology for Nurses and Health Visitors.* Macmillan, London.

Hanson, E. (1994) *The Cancer Nurse's Experience.* Quay Publications, Lancaster.

Hargie, O., Saunders, C., Dickson, D. (1994) *Social Skills in Interpersonal Communication.* Croom Helm, London.

Hearn, J., Higginson, I.J. (1998) 'Do specialist palliative care teams improve outcomes for cancer patients? A systematic literature review.' *Palliative Medicine,* 12: 317–322.

Hebblethwaite, M. (1991) 'Shall we pretend it isn't happening?' *Journal of Advances in Health and Nursing Care*, 1 (2): 75–92.

Hodgson, H. (2000) 'Does reflexology impact on cancer patients' quality of life?' *Nursing Standard*, 14 (31): 33–38.

Karrer, R. (1996) 'The Macmillan touch.' *Practice Nurse*, 11 (6): 377–382.

Kendrick, K.D. (1999) 'Challenging power, autonomy and politics in complementary therapies: a contentious view.' *Journal of Complementary Therapies in Nursing and Midwifery*, 5 (3): 77–81.

Kendrick, K.D., Kinsella, M. (1994) 'Beyond the veil: truth telling in palliative care.' *Journal of Cancer Care*, 3 (4): 211–215.

Kendrick, K.D., Shea, T. (1995) 'With velvet gloves: the ethics of collusion.' *Palliative Care Today*, 4 (1): 9–11.

Kendrick, K.D., Weir, P. (1996) 'Truth telling in palliative care: a nursing response.' In Soothill K., Henry, I.C., Kendrick, K.D. (eds) *Themes and Perspectives in Nursing*, 2e. Chapman and Hall, London.

Klagsburn, S.C. (1981) 'Hospice: a developing role.' In Saunders, C., Summers, D.H., Teller, N. (eds) *Hospice: the living idea*. WB Saunders, Philadelphia.

Krakauer, E.L. (1996) 'Attending to death: limitations of medical technology (a resident's perspective)'. In Spiro, H.M., McCrea Curnen, M.G., Palmer Wandel, L. (eds) *Facing Death: where culture, religion and medicine meet*. Yale University Press, London.

Levi, D.S. (1998) 'Is death a bad thing?' *Mortality*, 3(3): 229–250.

Maguire, P., Faulkner, A. (1993) 'Communicating with cancer patients 1. Handling bad news and difficult questions.' In Dickenson, D., Johnson, M. (1993) *Death, Dying and Bereavement*. Sage Publications, London, in association with The Open University, Milton Keynes.

Penson, J. (1991) 'Complementary therapies.' In Penson, J., Fisher, R. (eds) *Palliative Care for People with Cancer*. Arnold, London.

Porter, R. (1989) 'Death and the doctors in Georgian England.' In Houlbrooke, R. (ed) *Death, Ritual and Bereavement*. Routledge, London.

Rycroft-Malone, J., Latter, S., Yerrell, P., Shaw, D. (2000) 'Nursing and medication education.' *Nursing Standard*, 14 (50): 35–39.

Scott, G. (1995) 'Challenging conventional roles in palliative care.' *Nursing Times*, 91(3): 38–39.

Smith, R. (2000) 'A good death.' *British Medical Journal*, 320 (15 January): 129–130.

Walters, T. (1994) *The Revival of Death*. Routledge, London.

Woolf, F., Marsnik, N., Tracey, W., Nicols, R. (1983) *Perceptive Listening*. Holt, Rinehart & Winston, New York.

3 Deciding about Treatment: advance directives and the law

Case Study 3.1 John and his family

It is the moment we all fear, when the decision has to be made about how the medical team should treat the person we love. John was 78 and suffered from Alzheimer's disease. Formerly a professor of engineering, he had been an energetic man throughout his life until the condition overtook him. Above all, he had been very sharp intellectually, delighting in the cut and thrust of debate. Many times he had said to his wife and sons that he could not bear the thought of living like a shell. He did not want euthanasia but, in the event of a severe physical illness such as a heart attack or stroke, he would not want to be revived.

Now John's wife Grace, and sons Tim and Geoff, sat with a doctor in an anteroom and tried to focus on the fact the John had suffered a major stroke. Grace was simply too shocked and afraid to take things in. Tim the eldest son felt that he had to communicate the views of his father. 'Now is the time to let go', he said. 'He wouldn't want to be kept alive as a vegetable'. For him the last two years, seeing his father in nursing care, had been painful. John was not the father he knew. Geoff was less sure. He had come to understand a different side of his father in those years. Much of his life he had feared John's intellect and felt that he would never live up to the expectations put on him. Since his father had been in nursing care he had learned to communicate with him in a non-cognitive way and had been glad to care for him. If there was a chance that the effects of the stroke might be reversed he wanted to keep him.

The doctor was young, uncertain and had many other problems to face. She was unsure how to bring this to a resolution. 'I guess in the end that it comes down to what John actually wanted, how he would want to retain dignity'.

The voice which was absent from this discussion was, of course, that of John himself. Tim tried to articulate his father's voice, but Geoff felt he had discovered quite another in his relationship. Grace was too upset even to begin thinking about what he would have wanted. What difference would the written communication of John's voice have made to them?

The issue of so called 'living wills' is about the articulating of a voice at just such a time, about the patient finding a voice in the difficult and confused moments which surround such a decision. We shall return to this case at the end of the next chapter.

The whole area of living wills is confused. Forms of advance directives, communicating the patient's wishes about future treatment, have been used for over 20 years. There is, however, no standard form or legal framework for their use. The medical profession has at times been unsure about their use and usefulness, often associating it with euthanasia. This is not surprising, as voluntary euthanasia groups have taken great interest in this field. This association has tended to place the living will firmly on the margins, something reinforced by the advocacy of the Voluntary Euthanasia Society and the Terrence Higgins Trust. As Sommerville puts, it the living will has been perceived by many as 'the last resort of marginalised groups' (Sommerville 1996: 36). In fact most of the legal cases which have taken forward the debate about living wills have involved young people, notably Tony Bland (see page 53).

Recent surveys on living wills show that while the public view them as good practice, very few actually have one. One survey suggests that only 13 per cent of people have taken out a living will (Luttrell and Sommerville 1996).

As we shall see, the interest in living wills has been such over the past two decades that several countries have developed legislation and Britain has been looking closely at the possibility of legislating for different kinds of advance directive. It is therefore a good time to begin to examine the idea of the living will.

History

The way in which people who are mentally incapacitated might find their own voice, and be able to communicate their hopes, desires and specific refusal of treatment, has been a concern since the 1960s. The concept of a 'living will' first emerged in the USA through writings of Louis Kutner (1969), who argued that the legal trust established over property should be equally permissible and applicable to one's body. The key point underlying Kutner's view of living wills is the importance of consent or withholding consent to treatment, whatever the prospect of recovery. This focuses on the patient's autonomy, and as Kutner has it 'the individual's right to privacy' (Kutner 1969). The living will seeks to maintain such rights when patients are no longer competent to speak for themselves. It was not long before such principles became enshrined in law.

The first State legislation was the California Death Act of 1976. This allowed for a 'cooling off' period of 14 days before the any directive could apply, sought to guard against abuse, and required that advance declarations be renewed every five years. The Indiana Living Wills and Life Prolonging Procedures Act 1989, noted the possibility of patients specifying treatment as well as refusing it. Much of this thinking came together in the 1990 Federal Self Determination Act which requires health care centres to advise patients at the point of admission of their right to accept or refuse and to set out an advance directive. It also becomes the task of the centre to find out if the patient has an advance directive. Medicare or Medicaid reimbursement is conditional on compliance with the Act. This Act was developed in response to the case of *Curzan* v. *Director* in which the 14th Amendment, which guards against deprivation of life, liberty or property without due legal process, was seen to apply to the liberty of the competent patient to refuse medical treatment.

The Code of Federal Regulations (updated on October 1, 2001) sets out detailed requirements for health care providers, including:

- The need to document and register an advance directive in the patient's records
- The need to provide education for staff concerning the policies and procedures on advance directives

- The need to provide wide community education which emphasises that advance directives 'enhance an incapacitated individual's control over medical treatment' (US Government, Code of Federal Regulations, Title 42, Vol. 3, Part 489, (6) a).

Now all States have legislation for advance medical directives and also for proxy, someone who will speak on behalf of the patient if they are not competent. Many States have particular forms to register both functions. Many of these State forms also recognise the validity of forms from other States. While some are silent on this issue, the American Bar Association advises that if a form from one State fails to meet the legal requirements of another it should still be treated as important, 'if not controlling', evidence (ABA 2002). Increasingly the advice in America is to combine an advance directive with the appointment of a proxy. It is recognised that no advance directive can necessarily apply to all situations without interpretation, something that a proxy can help with. There is also a concern for the proper registration and storing of living wills and values leading to the development of various registries on the Internet, including the US Living Wills Registry (www.uslivingwillregistry.com).

The experience of America has, nonetheless, been ambiguous. There is an increase in choice for many patients. However, there have been real problems with the delivery of this right:

1 The statutory nature of the process has led to an increase in litigation. This in can lead to the danger of doctors being concerned primarily to avoid litigation and not to think through the most appropriate response.
2 Acutely ill patients were not always in a position to refer to living will documents when entering hospital, still less participate in rational discussion about their use (La Puma *et al.* 1991).
3 In practice the right to choose was not equally distributed. Patients on Medicare and Medicaid (State medical support) tended to be less able to articulate their wishes (Silva and Sorrell 1984). More broadly it was also found that those who read informed consent statements carefully tended to be white, better educated and younger.

In Canada there is a reliance on case law for the principle of patient's wishes taking precedence over the physicians (Molloy and Mepham

1990). In addition Nova Scotia and Quebec have recognised in law, proxy designations in health care, while Ontario and Manitoba have developed legislation for advance directives (Advance Directives Seminar Group 1992). Canada has also developed a central living wills registry.

Across Europe practices vary. A very advanced example is Denmark, which has legally recognised living wills since 1992. A brochure of details is available in libraries, chemists and doctors' surgeries. This includes a form for registration in Copenhagen University. Faced by someone who is in a critical condition the doctor has to contact the directory to see if there is a living will registered.

The position in Ireland is much less clear. It is possible to set out views regarding future medical care. However, there is no legislation on living wills. The legal context, obviously, requires that any living will relate to lawful treatment (Costello 2000). The Supreme Court (in *re a Ward of Court*, 27 July 1995) upheld an earlier High Court judgement consenting to the withdrawal and termination of artificial means of feeding in the case of a ward of court in near permanent vegetative state, on the application of the family. John Costello notes that this ruling suggests that views expressed by a person about future medical treatment would be referred to by the court in coming to any decision about the withdrawal of treatment. However, Costello concludes, 'the context in which these views relate and the extent to which they are binding on medical professionals remains unclear' (Costello 2000: 161). Hence, any concerns about living wills, from health care practitioners or patients, should be referred to a solicitor.

The United Kingdom

In the UK in recent years there have been a number of important debates and documents about living wills and the surrounding issues of mental capacity and definition of care.

1 In 1988 the Report *The Living Will: Consent to Treatment at the End of Life* was published. The working party, chaired by Ian Kennedy, and subsequent report was under the auspices of the Age Concern Institute of Gerontology and the Centre of Medical Law and Ethics, Kings College London.

2 In 1994 the House of Lords Select Committee on Medical Ethics examined this area calling amongst other things for a code of practice on advance directives for health professionals.

3 A code was produced in 1995 by the BMA, *Advance Statements about Medical Treatment*. In 1996 The Patients Association produced a guide for patients, *Advance Statements about Future Medical Treatment*.

4 The Law Commission's report on *Mental Incapacity* was published in 1995.

5 This was followed 1997 by a Consultation Paper, *Who Decides? Making Decisions on behalf of Mentally Incapacitated Adults* (Lord Chancellor's Department 1997).

6 This has resulted in the report from the Government, *Making Decisions* (Lord Chancellor's Office 1999), which will form the basis for legislation.

7 1999 also saw the publication by the Scottish Executive of '*Making the Right Moves*' (Scottish Executive 1999). This formed the basis for the subsequent Adults with Incapacity (Scotland) Act, 2000, which is referred to in more detail below.

As we shall see these debates have served to refine our understanding of the different issues involved in advance directives but have not led to a demand for any actual legislation.

Defining terms

The very terms used can be confusing, ranging from 'living wills' to 'advance statements' and 'advance directives', sometimes referring to slightly different approaches, often used interchangeably (Holt 2002) . The term 'living will' itself is confusing, not least because it does not refer to post mortem communication, is not legally binding, and is not a mechanism of distributing resources. In its place, many authorities prefer to use the overall term 'advance statements', and these can be divided into three categories of ways in which patients who are not competent to make a decision can find a voice:

- Values histories
- Proxy decisions
- Advance directives.

Values statements or histories

These may involve:

- A simple statement that reflects the person's hope and preferences in terms of treatment. This is not binding on the health care team but can be a helpful part of the decision making process.
- A values history. This provides information about the person's belief and values. As the Scottish Euthanasia Society notes, this is not about how individuals want to die as much as how they may want to live until they die.

A values history examines:

- The important relationships
- How the person feels about dependence and independence
- The person's views of death and suffering
- The person's belief system and spirituality
- The person's views of health and illness.

In effect, the values history enables patients to articulate their story. There is no suggestion that such statements should be part of any legislation.

Proxy decisions

One well-tried approach to the communication of the views of the patient is through proxy, i.e. a person who is close to the patient and appointed to speak as a 'surrogate' on the patient's behalf. Many American States encourage this approach alongside advance directives. The surrogate can assist with the interpretation of the directive, overcoming possible ambiguities and assisting in the decision making process.

In English law, there is nothing to prevent patients appointing someone to act as their agent for medical decisions. However, such appointments are revoked automatically once the commissioning person is no longer competent to make them (Montgomery 1994). The Enduring Power of Attorney Act 1985 enables the appointment of persons to administer the property of the person who is mentally incompetent, but this does not apply to medical decisions (McHale and Fox 1997:883). At this stage the powers that apply to property do not extend in law to decisions about welfare or consent for medical treatment.

Advance directives

Advance directives are what most people mean when they refer to 'living wills', and we will use this term from now on. This involves a specific recorded direction from the patient indicating the refusal of some or all of medical treatment. Made by a competent adult, this can have legal force. An advance directive acknowledges that advance refusal is as valid as a contemporaneous refusal of treatment. A medical practitioner is bound to comply when the directive specifically addresses the medical situation that has arisen. Since no-one can actually demand specific treatment, then advance directives are by definition refusals.

We will now examine these three categories in more detail.

Values histories

The values history is in many respects the least contentious way of communicating the patient's wishes. Firstly, the history can take many forms, from a story format, to a dialogue, to a pre-set form with different category headings. This is precisely because it uses the language of the person involved, thus it is less likely to marginalise those with limited knowledge of the medical field or those whose first language is not English. As we saw above, the American experience of 'advance directives' was quite the opposite.

Secondly, values histories are less open to the possible criticism of not being established at the time of writing. There is no question of having to be certain about the competence of the patient and in particular whether she actually understood treatments, medical conditions or states, and their consequences. There is also then no attempt to speculate about future states and how the person might feel about those states.

Thirdly, values histories are essentially person centred and therefore focus on the autonomy of the person in terms of the basic values and preferences. This gives a broader approach to decision making than simply the refusal. In effect this enables the person to clarify her own values and principles and thus enables those values to become part of the decision making process. Emmanuel and Emmanuel see this is a critical part of the development of autonomy:

'Freedom and control over medical decisions alone do not constitute patient autonomy. Autonomy requires that individuals
critically assess their own values and preferences; determine
whether they are desirable; affirm, upon reflection, these values as
ones which justify their actions; and then be free to initiate action
which will realise those values.' (Emanuel and Emanuel
1992:2225)

In this light it may be argued that the broader view of the person and
values is more important than any specific medical directive. Such
medical data has its problems, as we shall see.

Fourthly, the experience of the American directives suggested that
advance directives were not enduring and that they should be rewrit-
ten every five years. The values history too may need reflection and
revision, but it is by definition more enduring. It provides core values
that will be less likely to change over time.

Fifthly, the values history detracts from a focus on the law and how the
patient and doctor have to adhere to the conditions of the law. This
then focuses on the situation in hand and how the most creative decision can be made.

Sixthly, it is not constrained to a few situations but can rather be
applied to a wide range of situations.

Seventhly, it helps to understand the patient as a person and not simply
as an object in a medico–legal dialogue. Hence, we can get away from
the atmosphere of fear found in such contexts. The health care professional can easily raise the idea of values history in a positive way that can
inform the whole of the patient's treatment. In this way, it is not simply
associated with death situations. Equally this provides an important
focus for dialogue between the medical profession and patients. There is
a strong argument for including this as a regular part of care delivery,
enabling patients to build up over time a real appreciation of their values
and of how these relate to illness and suffering. In the next chapters we
will examine in more detail how the values history can become a means
of value clarification, and how this can affect patient autonomy.

Finally, the values history is a way of avoiding the problems of too
much detail in directives. As one writer puts it, 'the more detailed an

advance directive is, the more likely it is to vary from events that actually occur' (Dickens 1993:80).

Even where an advance directive is used, values history would make a good addition enabling creative decision making. The Canadian Medical Association Seminar Group on Advance Directives (1992) suggests that:

> 'Since values and preferences represent fundamentally different but complementary approaches, instruction directives should contain both of these components.' (Advance Directives Seminar Group 1992:129)

The values history then recognises that decision making is best made when the person knows something about the patient. Often these beliefs and values are best expressed in narrative form. It is less threatening to the clinical judgement of the doctor than advance directives and offers a real basis for decision making that involves next of kin and medical staff, all of whom appear comfortable with this idea. At the same time the process of value history taking and sharing is one that challenges the doctor to integrate personal as well as medical factors into decision making.

Proxy

The Law Commission proposed that an individual should be able to produce a treatment proxy, extending the enduring power of attorney (EPA). At present there are two types of attorney. The ordinary power of attorney lasts for as long as the 'donor' (the person who gives the power) retains mental capacity. This power is used, for instance, when a person goes abroad for some time and wants their affairs handled at home. The second extends this through the EPA Act 1985 to the time when the donor is mentally incapacitated, and applies to property. The present system has many potential problems:

- Family members may not know about the existence of the EPA
- In some cases the donor was already mentally incapacitated when they signed the EPA
- There has been no adequate provision to ensure that the registration of the EPA is completed once the donor has lost his or her capacity to take decisions

- The court will not know about an unregistered power being exercised
- The rigid insistence on the use of a form makes it much less flexible than advance directives.

These point to the possibility of abuse or neglect, even under the present Act.

In the USA the trend is towards proxy legislation for medical decisions, along with advance directive, used simply to guide the decision (Age Concern Institute of Gerontology 1988:68). In English law there is no recognition of the idea of 'substituted judgement' – the surrogate taking a decision that the patient would have made in that situation (*Airedale NHS* v. *Bland*). Hence, the principle of judgement is in the first place to try to find unequivocal evidence of the patient's wishes, and failing this to apply the principle of best interest.

For and against

The extension of the power of attorney to medical decisions is attractive for several reasons. Firstly, it allows for flexible response to the particular situation. The proxy decision maker can take into account changing circumstances. Secondly, the proxy may be more available than an advance directive, which may be stored some way away. Thirdly, research suggests that the majority of patients prefer to place their trust in someone speaking for them rather than simply a written advance directive (High 1993; Sam and Singer 1993). Finally, while the advance directive makes a contribution to the decision making process it does enable the dialogue that allows the person to really confront the issues of mortality.

Ranged against these themes are four arguments. Firstly, a significant number of people may not have anyone they can ask to be a proxy, or may find it hard to choose one. Furthermore the choice of proxy may become out of date (McHale 1998:326). A person acceptable originally may no longer be so. Secondly, there is danger of proxies being ignored or not used. Thirdly, when faced by the challenge of having to make a decision the proxy, especially if he or she is close to the patient, may not be emotionally capable of carrying out the patient's wishes. Emmanuel and Emmanuel (1993) conclude this of two thirds of proxies. For many people the decision to refuse treatment is seen in itself as a betrayal of the patient. Finally, statistically significant research shows that proxies may have no better than an average understanding of the patient's wishes. Medical staff fare little better; Emmanuel and Emmanuel (1993) conclude advance directives would more clearly and accurately communicate the wishes of the patient. There is also the danger that the proxy might not apply the criteria that the patient set out. Evidence suggests that those close to patients tend to err towards a more general concern for their best interest, usually resuscitation (Seckler 1991).

Montgomery sees the use of proxy as a form of paternalism that overrules the autonomy of the patient. If then the proxy is to take fully into account the wishes of the patient there needs to be a careful legal framework (Montgomery 1994).

The Government's response

In examining this the Government has concluded that proxy is an important element in ensuring the voice of the patient and that it should be placed in such a framework. The UK Government intends to extend the Enduring Power of Attorney to a Continuing Power of Attorney (CPA). This would both address the difficulties of the EPA and take into account the needs with respect to healthcare decision making.

Continuing Powers of Attorney

'The Government intends to put in place a system of CPAs that would enable a person to delegate decision making powers on finance, healthcare and personal welfare, where both donor and donee are over 18.' (Lord Chancellor's Office 1999:2.4).

With respect to healthcare this would not allow the attorney to make any decisions about treatment unless the donor 'is, or is reasonably believed to be, without capacity' (2.3). Nor could the donee give consent to compulsory treatment of the donor under the Mental Health Act 1983.

The attorney would not be able to consent to the withdrawal of artificial nutrition and hydration without specific authority to do so stated in the CPA. General authority to make decisions could not extend to such actions. The use of the healthcare power would not be permitted until the donor is incapacitated.

The Government White Paper *Making Decisions* (Lord Chancellor's Office 1999) is also careful to make clear that certain decisions could never be part of the CPA, including consent to marriage, divorce, sexual relations, adoption and decisions about voting for elections to public office.

Safeguards

Given this scope, the Government then looks to set in place safeguards. The aim of the safeguards is to provide protection of those without capacity, while at the same time trying to minimise interference where relationships are good and care is successful. These safeguards cover the making of CPAs, and procedures, including registration and safeguards against abuse:

1 The form for a CPA would be prescribed, with its terms set out in writing. This will be signed, dated and witnessed. The form should be accompanied by evidence that the donor was competent at the time of its completion. This could involve either a medical certificate or a signed statement by the donor's doctor as part of the form. Donors will be able to appoint more than one attorney either to deal with different decisions or to make joint decisions. Similarly, substitute attorneys will be able to be appointed in case the earlier appointees lose their mental capacity or die. The donee has to be a particular person and not the holder of a specific office. As noted above, the power to make certain decisions can only be given if specified in the CPA.

2 While they have mental capacity, donors will be able to revoke or amend the CPA, or change attorney. Equally the attorney can withdraw consent to act under a CPA. Selecting someone to act as attorney in the context outlined above is a very personal matter, involving a high degree of trust. Because of this, if the original attorney is unable or unwilling to fulfil this role, and if there is no substitute attorney, the court will not be able to appoint a substitute

attorney. However, the court will be able to appoint a manager, as an agent for the person who is mentally incapable and who will be subject to stricter control than the attorney.

3 There will be a compulsory registration system and a Registering Authority. The CPA must be registered before attorneys can use their power. This authority can check whether other persons are registered for the same person. If there are problems in this it can refer to the courts for a ruling. Registration will be possible from the execution of CPA up to the time when the donor become incapable of making decisions. Financial and welfare matters can be handled by the donee while the donor is still capable, if that is the donor's wish. However, healthcare matters can only be dealt with by donees when donors lose their mental capacity. This enables attorneys to take up the powers immediately in the event of sudden traumatic incapacity of the donor.

4 The Government proposes that the notification of relevant others about the application for registration of the CPA should take place before registration. This would enable any disputes and challenges to this application to be addressed by the courts prior to the CPA becoming effective. It is recommended that a period of 28 days should elapse between notification and registration to allow for any objections to be lodged with the Registering Authority.

All this would be under the Court of Protection, and would also include measures to protect the attorney from any liability.

The detailed attention given to this section by the Government demonstrates the importance of this to the matter of communicating the patient's view in any decision about treatment. Not only would it broaden the scope of the Power of Attorney, it would also ensure that real safeguards for the process are set in place. The proposed legislation also would ensure ways of speedily enabling the proper authorities to recognise the status of attorneys, enabling them to make decisions effectively, and at the appropriate time (2.6).

Managers

Making Decisions (Lord Chancellor's Office 1999) also proposes that, if an attorney is unable or unwilling to continue to perform their duties on behalf of the donor, then the court (Court of Protection) will not be able to appoint a substitute attorney. The logic behind this is that the choice of a attorney on the part of the donor is highly personal and built upon trust. The court could not hope to make a similar appointment on behalf of the mentally incapacitated patient. However, the court would be able to appoint a manager subject to stricter control than an attorney. Several requirements will apply to all managers:

- The manager will be obliged to act in the best interest of the person without capacity
- The manager must be an individual over the age of 18 or a trust corporation (in relation to property or financial matters)
- The manager can be the holder of a specific office, provided there is no conflict of interest
- More than one manager can be appointed
- The manager will be regarded in law as a statutory agent for the person without capacity
- Managers can do nothing that is not consistent with an attorney acting within their authority.

The manager would have the power to deal with:

- The control and management of any property, and its disposal or acquisition
- The carrying out of any business, trade or profession
- Dissolution of any partnership
- Carrying out of any contract
- Discharge of any debt or obligation (Lord Chancellor's Office 1999:3.24).

Several groups argue that managers ought to have the power to refuse consent to healthcare. However, because such decisions tend to be 'one-off' the Government counters that there is no need to appoint a manager for these, rather they should be settled by the court. This includes the issue of withdrawal of 'artificial nutrition and hydration' for a person in a persistent vegetative state (PVS).

All of this demands the setting up of a new single court jurisdiction, to be based in the Court of Protection. The court would be able to remove any manager who, it felt, was not acting in the best interest of the patient or was in some way unsuitable.

Underlying the Government's work on proxies and managers is a concern to ensure proper patient advocacy.

At the time of writing there has been no confirmed timetable for this legislation.

Age Concern supports the proposal for Continuing Power of Attorney and, in a policy position paper on capacity and consent, argues that it should be referred to as Registered Power of Attorney to ensure that there is no confusion about when it can be used (Age Concern England 2002).

Advance directives

In the UK there is no legal statute on advance directives. Nonetheless, advance directives (refusals) are recognised in common law. Three particular cases have established this precedent, in terms of doctors being bound by consent.

These were set in the English courts and have been thought to apply throughout the UK. Devolution has affected legislation, with the development of the Adults with Incapacity (Scotland) Act 2000 (see page 61). This, however, legislates for welfare attorneys and not for advance directives.

Case Study 3.2 Re T [1992] 4 All E.R.649

A woman in late pregnancy, Miss T, was involved in a road accident. Three days later she was admitted to hospital and treated for pneumonia. The next day Miss T began the first stages of labour, while still suffering the symptoms of pneumonia. She signed a form refusing her consent for a blood transfusion, without considering alternative treatment. In the event she had a caesarean section without needing blood transfusion, although the baby was stillborn. Her condition then deteriorated, and it was determined that she would die without a blood transfusion.

The Court of Appeal had to determine whether her refusal was legally valid; whether she had been unduly influenced in her decision and whether the patient had a right to refuse invasive treatment that might be otherwise imposed on them in the future. The Court of Appeal unanimously decided that the doctors had a right to give the blood transfusion partly because the relevant treatment options were not made clear to her, and partly because it was felt that her mother, a Jehovah's Witness, had had undue influence upon her. The patient herself was not a practising Jehovah's Witness. However, in terms of the advance treatment the Court established the principle that where an informed and capable patient makes a choice 'which is clearly established and applicable in the circumstances', medical staff would be bound by it, just as they would be bound by a contemporaneous refusal of treatment.

Lord Donaldson noted, '*Prima facie* every adult has the right and capacity to decide whether or not he will accept medical treatment even if a refusal may risk permanent injury to his health or even lead to premature death'.

Case Study 3.3 Airedale NHS Trust v. Bland

Tony Bland was a victim of the Hillsborough Football disaster in which 95 supporters were killed due to the effects of overcrowding in the 1989 semi-final of the FA Cup. Bland suffered severe crush injuries and was subsequently left in a persistent vegetative state (PVS).

Medical opinion was unanimous on the diagnosis and that there was no hope of recovery, and the result of the legal case was that tube feeding was withdrawn.

Lord Bingham summed up the principles that both parties agreed on:

'It is a civil wrong and may be a crime to impose medical treatment on a conscious adult of sound mind without his or her consent'. Hence 'a medical practitioner must comply with clear instructions given by an adult of sound mind as to the treatment given or not given in certain circumstances, whether these instructions are rational or irrational. This principle applies even if, by the time the specific circumstances pertain, the patient is unconscious or no longer of sound mind'.

Lord Goff is even more specific, concluding, 'It has been held that a patient of sound mind may, if properly informed, require that life support be discontinued. The same principle applies where the patient's refusal to give his consent has been expressed at an earlier date, before he became unconscious or otherwise incapable of communicating it'.

Lords Musthill, Goff and Keith all accepted that health care professionals would be guilty of battery if they treated someone who had given an advance directive refusing treatment. This does not mean that doctors are always compelled to work according to the contents of an advanced directive. They would have to consider its scope and applicability to the situation in hand.

Case Study 3.4 Re C (Adult Refusal of Treatment) [1994] 1 ALL ER8 19

A patient in Broadmoor hospital suffered the delusion that he was medically qualified. He developed a gangrenous infection in one leg, and the consultant surgeon estimated that he would have a 15 per cent chance of survival without amputation. C refused consent for the amputation. In the event, more conservative care was accepted by C and he survived without amputation. However, the surgeon believed that C's leg might deteriorate and become life-threatening in the future. As a result, C's solicitor sought a declaration from the court that no amputation would take place in the future without written consent. The High Court upheld this, holding the refusal from the patient be valid both for the present and in the future.

Building on this finding was a test of capacity set down by the Law Commission. This had a therapeutic threshold and a functional test. The threshold concerned those who were not able to make a decision due to 'mental instability'. This was defined as 'a disability or disorder of the mind or brain, whether permanent or temporary, which results in an impairment or disturbance of mental functioning' (McHale 1998, 322).

The functional test based on the ruling in Re C asked whether the person could comprehend and retain the information given to him or her, whether the person believed the information and whether they used the information to arrive at a choice (McHale 1998, 322). A person would lack capacity if he or she was unable to comprehend or retain the relevant data, and was thus unable to make use of it in making a decision.

In this case, the law found it irrelevant whether the directive contradicted the views of others including the medical establishment. The important point was that the person, C, was able to decide on the matter in question, even if he lacked insight into other aspects of his life. The patient in this case then was capable of making a decision about *this* issue, and not necessarily capable of making decision about all issues. Hence, incapacity was not to be equated with irrationality. This ruling was critical to the legal definition of capacity.

The BMA (1995) Code of Practice helpfully sums up the test of capacity (see Appendix I). To demonstrate capacity individuals should be able to:

- Understand in broad terms and simple language what the medical treatment is, its purpose and nature and why it is being proposed for them

- Understand its principal benefits, risks and alternatives
- Understand in broad terms what will be the consequences of not receiving the proposed treatment
- Make a free choice
- Retain the information long enough to make an effective decision (BMA 1995:26–27).

In all this the assessment of the person's capacity should be made in relation to the particular treatment proposed. There is also the presumption of capacity until the contrary is demonstrated. Capacity may vary over time if the patient is mentally disordered and thus health carers should identify and use the times when the patient is most capable. All assessment of capacity should be recorded in that person's medical notes.

Assessing capacity can be a complex matter. Some patients do not wish to know the full extent of their problem and thus may not have a real grasp of the implications of treatment. This can make it difficult for the doctor to ascertain whether the person fully understands the implications of the treatment.

Criteria for valid advance directives

Linda Wilson sums up the result of these three cases in terms of the criteria for advance directives to be valid:

- The person who has drawn up the advance directive must have been mentally competent, not suffering from any mental distress and over 18 when he or she made the request.
- The person must have been fully informed about the nature and consequence of the advance directive when he or she made it.
- The person made it clear that the advance directive should apply to all situations or circumstances that may arise at a later date.
- The person must not have been pressurised or influenced by anyone else when he or she made the advance directive.
- The advance directive has not been changed, either verbally or in writing, since it was drawn up.
- The person is now incapable of making any decisions because he or she is unconscious or otherwise unfit (Wilson 1999:6).

Treatment response

At the core of any treatment given by doctors is the right of the patient to refuse treatment for any reason, rational or irrational, even if that decision might lead to death. The performance 'of physically invasive treatment without the patient's consent is a criminal or tortuous assault' (Lord Chancellor's Department 1997:4.3). Treatment can be given, in the patient's best interests, to preserve life or to prevent deterioration in health, providing that this is not contrary to previous competent and valid expression of the patient's views.

This may involve clear directives, such as the refusal to have blood transfusions. It may not be easy, however, for two reasons. Firstly, the directive may not be precise enough to fit the treatment. Secondly, there may have been advances in treatments that a patient who made the directive several years earlier had not contemplated or understood (Jeffrey 2001:99).

In addition, doctors are not bound by the statements or patient wishes requiring them to do anything that is not lawful. This includes any attempts primarily to end the patient's life. Both the Law Commission and the Government are clear that there is no connection between advance statements and euthanasia, where the prime intention is to end the person's life. The Government has made it quite clear that there are no plans to change the law on euthanasia and that this would remain an offence of murder. Hence, there are no legal grounds for seeing such connections.

An advance directive is also superseded if it comes into conflict with existing statutes, in particular in mental health law. The Mental Health Act 1983 and the Mental Health (Scotland) Act 1984 both authorise treatment or care without consent in the interests of the patient's health and safety, and for the protection of other people. Any advance directive that refuses treatment for mental illness would be rendered invalid if the patient were legally detained for treatment under these statutes.

Best interest

Concern for the patient's best interest is not necessarily to be seen as a paternalistic stance. The Law Commission felt that best interest should include the patients' past and present wishes and feelings and the factors they might consider. This would then ensure that patients' wishes are routinely taken into account, and thus be part of defining their own individual best interest. Age Concern advocate the use of the term 'personal best interest' precisely for this reason (Age Concern England 2002).

The best interest criteria would ensure that patients would not be deprived of new treatments of which they had been unaware:

> 'The advance statement is not, therefore, to be seen in isolation, but against the background of the doctor/patient dialogue and the involvement of other carers who might be able to give an insight into what the patient would want in the particular circumstances of the case.' (Lord Chancellor's Department 1997:4)

While children do not have the same legal rights as adults, and under the age of 18 cannot make a valid advance directive, it is nonetheless important to include them in any decision making and to keep them fully informed about treatment options. The Children Act 1989 stresses that minors should be consulted about matters affecting their welfare. How this might be achieved is once more down to good relationships between the patient, doctor and family and friends. In the context of a trusting relationship it might be possible to take a narrative form of values history.

Care

The basic legal principle at the heart of directives is to do with autonomy in its negative form, that is, unless consent is given to treatment this is seen as an assault on the person. This does not mean that there is an overriding principle of self-determination in all aspects of the treatment. Hence the BMA guidelines note that, where there is a directive refusing basic care and maintenance of the non-competent patient, this should not be binding on the carers.

The law does not provide clear guidelines on this matter. However, while the consent of the patient remains critical, any refusal should be set aside in the exceptional circumstances that this causes harm to others or places an intolerable burden on the carers. In the first of these it may be that lack of attention to the care and hygiene of the patient could lead to infection that could affect others. In the second category, if the patient is not made comfortable or free of pain this could makes things difficult to bear for the family and medical staff.

Where there is a directive that is against all interventions on the part of the medical team, the BMA guidelines suggest that this should rule out all but measures essential to patient comfort. Such basic care includes:

- Provision of warmth and shelter
- Management of symptoms that distress the patient such as breathlessness and vomiting
- Hygiene control, such as managing incontinence.

These express respect for the dignity of individual patients, in whatever condition they find themselves. Towards the end of life, nutrition and hydration become less important for the patient, but even this does not rule out moistening the patient's lips to provide coolness and comfort.

To balance this, while appropriate food and drink should be made available it should not be forced upon the person. Where there is an advance refusal of tube feeding this should be respected.

Once again it comes back down to finding the right balance, and this means going beyond the law to the relationship which the health care team has with the patient at whatever stage. At its heart, this is about expressing respect for the patient.

There is real difficulty in the whole process of knowing precisely what constitutes 'acceptable care'. The law does not give guidance on this. It is critical for practitioners to be able to act safely, according to the basic level of care in this situation, not least because they can be subject to accusations of negligence.

Pregnancy

The case of Re S [1992] 4 All E.R. 671 centred on the refusal of a pregnant woman to consent to a caesarean section. The High Court overruled this and allowed the operation to be performed. This case has not been helpful in that it appears to conflict with the later case, Re C (see Case 3.4, featured earlier in this chapter). Many respondents to the Law Commission (1995) document and to *Who Decides?* (Lord Chancellor's Department 1997) argue that this would subject the woman to 'unlawful battery'. It may be possible to justify such intervention from the courts where there is a viable fetus that may be in danger. As McHale and Fox (1997:876) note this ruling also illustrates that there is no absolute right to die.

The majority of US states suspend any advance directives during pregnancy, precisely because of the special status of the fetus, but also because this may involve a different situation from that envisaged in the directive itself.

The Law Commission and the Government are both concerned that the woman's right to determine what happens to her body should not 'evaporate' simply because of pregnancy. However, the Law Commission also recommended that the advance refusal should only apply if the woman had specified it as covering pregnancy. This still does not deal with all problem areas. It would certainly rule out all generalised refusals. However, at the same time a woman might have made an advance refusal that specifies no consent to caesarean sections, viewing this in the context of labour. In certain situations, however, this operation may be necessary to save the life of the woman or the child or both. The law in relation to this runs the danger of being a blunt instrument and cannot be a substitute for careful reflection that takes into account the context of the directive and the context of the present situation.

The Law Commission noted that, where there was doubt, life should be preserved, with the refusal being presumed not to apply. This was further refined with the view that, where the refusal of treatment might lead to death, this should be explicitly stated in the advance refusal for it to be valid.

Liability of health care providers

If treatment, which is against a clearly communicated valid advance directive, is carried out, there is always the danger of a health care provider being found guilty of battery. However, the Law Commission helpfully clarifies the existing law by noting that where a health care professional either withdraws treatment in accordance with the patient's wish as he or she understood it, or proceeded with treatment when, unknown to the practitioner the patient had directed otherwise, the professional should not incur liability in the law of tort (as in trespass to the person). Critically, it would be the responsibility of the person who has made an advance refusal to ensure that this was communicated to the health care professional.

Scotland

As noted above the Scottish Executive has also been working through to legislation in this area. *Making the Right Moves* (Scottish Executive 1999) set down proposed legislation which takes account of the fact the principle of best interest enshrined in the English legislation would not be binding in Scotland. This has led to the Adults with Incapacity (Scotland) Act 2000.

This also refuses to legislate for advance directives, for the same reasons:

'Attempts to legislate in this area will not adequately cover all situations which might arise, and could produce unintended and undesirable results in individual cases.' (Scottish Executive 1999, 6.14)

Section 5 of the legislation seeks to ensure that the doctor will consult with family, 'guardian', 'welfare attorney' or person authorised under an intervention order. Where there is disagreement it will be referred to a nominated medical practitioner, who will also consult the relevant persons. In the light of further disagreement it will be referred to the Court of Session. Section 1 also confirms that all attempts should be made to take account of: 'the present and past wishes and feelings of the adult so far as they can be ascertained by any means of communication, whether human or by mechanical aid (whether interpretative or otherwise) appropriate to the adult' (Scottish Executive 1999, Part 1, 1, 4 (a)).

The necessary changes in practice include a strengthening of the office of Public Guardian. The Public Guardian's tasks will include supervision of guardian or authorised person, maintenance of registers, and receipt and investigation of any complaints about the exercise of guardian functions in relation to property and finance. The grant of power of attorney is open to inspection and may be challenged. In such cases the Sheriff's court is able to terminate the grant to protect the interest of the incapable person.

The grant of power of attorney must comply with basic conditions:

- It should be in written form and witnessed
- It should clearly state the power granted
- The person must be 16 years of age or over
- It should include a certificate from a solicitor confirming that the person understands the role and process and is not acting under 'undue influence'.

European Legislation

The Human Rights Act 1998 incorporates into UK law the European Convention on Human Rights. Under Article 2 of the Convention a person's rights are to be protected by law. Article 3 prohibits inhuman and degrading treatment. Article 8 requires respect for private and family life. As these articles are tested in case law the exact application of the rights will become clear. What case law there is confirms that existing principles of common law are consistent with the Convention [A National Health Trust v. D (2000) 55BMLR 19; NHS Trust A v. M and NHS Trust B v. H (2000) 58 BMLR 87]. In the case of D v. UK (1997) EHRR 423 the European Court held that Article 3 includes the right to die with dignity. Given this weight of legal interest it is likely that the response of healthcare professionals will be subject to greater scrutiny, and thus the decision making process will need to be open, transparent and justifiable.

Summary

We can begin to sum up the major arguments for and against advance directives.

Arguments for

1 The advance directive provides reassurance for patients who fear that the continued application of life saving technology may deny their dignity.

2 It protects patient autonomy, providing the closest we can get to the relevant decision any individual person would have made.

3 It can stimulate and focus the doctor-patient dialogue, ensuring that the patient's voice is included in medical decision making.

4 Through expressing the detailed concerns of an individual, the advance directive can reduce ambiguity.

5 Provided the use of advance directives is made clear, they can provide both guidance and legal protection for medical staff.

6 Advance directives ease the emotional burden of the family, ensuring they do not have to be responsible for life and death decisions.

Arguments against

1 It is difficult to simply apply a pre-determined wish to a situation that has yet to happen and which therefore lacks any data. Inevitably in the light of a situation there will be different interpretations of the statements. Importantly, this means that interpretation and judgement of those involved at the time remains vital. Minimally, the doctor, other medical staff and family have to be sure that the directive fulfils the criteria of competence.

2 The patient may have a change of mind before the event, but not get round to changing the directive. This is particularly problematic if the patient is relying totally on the advance directive, without having a continued dialogue with a specific medical practitioner.

3 The actual scenario may be very different from the one envisaged by the patient. It may include, for instance, newly developed technology that may alleviate the situation in ways not envisaged when the directive was made.

4 There is the danger of creating a 'slippery slope', a situation in which directives will be used to save scarce health care resources, and people even encouraged to make them for that reason. This will be examined more closely in the next chapter.

5 There is the possibility that patients may not understand complex forms. The American experience has shown that less articulate people can be disadvantaged by this approach.

6 The advance directive does not enable full reflection on the core life values of the patient.

7 It has been argued, especially from religious sources, that the advance directive takes away both from the sanctity of life and the sovereignty of God. In effect the refusal of treatment may lead to death and this cannot be accepted as a consequence of refusal of treatment.

8 Patients may not understand treatments or be able to distinguish them from palliative care.

9 Advance directives that embody a patient's specific wishes as a legal right run the risk of never succeeding in those terms. If the directive is too precise, it might be hard to find exact applicability. If it is too broad, it loses any content in terms of the wishes of the patient with regard to treatment.

10 Without proper safeguards there is the danger that advance directives could be used with the intent of ending the patient's life. This, again, may have the 'slippery slope' effect. The more that advance directives are simply accepted the more we may accept that the consequence of the directive is death and the more it is viewed as intending death.

The legal foundation

Of a different order to the arguments against the advance directive above is the one that questions the generally accepted view of case law as providing a basis for them.

In the case of Bland it was stated that 'At no time before the disaster did Mr Bland give any indication of his wishes should he find himself in such a condition' (Lord Goff). In this light, any comments on advance directives by the judges are *obiter*, i.e. not directly in issue in the case before them thus neither requiring a decision nor setting a binding legal precedent. At the most such comments have a persuasive authority, which should, of course be taken into account in future decisions. In the case of Re T, the key issue was whether the patient's mother had undue influence on her. While this has relevance to the question of competence, it does not involve an advance directive *per se*.

In the case of Re C, it is important to note that the patient was found not to be incapacitated. The Court found him to be competent and upheld and safeguarded his continued refusal. Once again, while this has real relevance to the issue of competence, it does not directly rule on advance directives (SPUC 1998:2.6).

The conclusion of such arguments is that, while case law provides some important insights into aspects that are relevant to advance directives, it cannot be seen as giving full legal weight to them. A much more modest conclusion of this case law was reached by the Official Solicitor in a Practice Note of 26 July 1996:

> 'The High Court may determine the effect of a purported advance directive as to future medical treatment: Re T (Adult: Refusal of Medical Treatment) Fam 95, sub nom; Re T (An Adult) (Consent to medical Treatment) [1994] 2FLR 458; Re C (Refusal of Medical Treatment) [1994] 1FLR31. In summary, the patient's previously expressed views, if any, will always be an important component in the decisions of the doctors and the court, particularly if those views are clearly established and were intended to apply to the circumstances which have in fact arisen.'

The legal position on advance directives then, is not simple. It recognises and supports the principles of consent to treatment while stopping short of unqualified support. It is precisely because of this that the Government in *Making Decisions* has concluded that it does not wish to introduce legislation on advance directives *per se*. It is concerned both to reinforce the underlying principles, such as consent to treatment, and also to encourage the right decision making practice in respect of the patient's wishes and the most appropriate treatment. Hence, it stresses the importance of working within the guidelines set down by the BMA, and has focused any legal changes on clarifying and strengthening the law on proxy and management. Where there is conflict, the Government believes it is better resolved in the courts. This is addressed by the Lord Chancellor in a speech to a Law Society Conference (Irvine of Lairg 1999:6):

> 'The courts have a great advantage over any possible statute. They can provide an individual assessment of the applicability of an advance statement, based on the individual circumstances of each

case. No statute could do that, however complex. Unless the legislation were to say that all disputes over advance statements must be resolved in court, the legislation would risk making advance statements inappropriate and inflexible, with the obvious dangers to the best interests of individuals which that would involve.'

Age Concern remain opposed to this view, arguing that regulation should lie in statute rather than common law: 'because acting on statements often happens at times of great stress to individuals and legislation makes the situation clearer for all parties concerned' (Age Concern England 2002).

A conclusion at this stage then about the different forms of advance statement is that they can play an important part in ensuring that the patient's wishes are fully informed and recognised. This means that all three approaches can be used together, to provide a voice for the patient. Finding such a voice, however, focuses increasingly on the need for good practice and the right process to encourage dialogue in treatment. Such good practice will enable the right context for the advance statement to be used most effectively.

However, before we can begin to look in more detail at what constitutes good practice, it is important to address some of the key ethical issues that have been bubbling up beneath the legal arguments. The conflict between paternalism and autonomy, for instance, sets up an important adversarial dynamic that underlies the legal debate. We must now examine this and other ethical debates more closely to see precisely what are the key principles of advance directives.

References

Advance Directives Seminar Group (1992) 'Advance Directives: Are they an advance?' *Canadian Medical Association Journal*, 146 (2).

Age Concern England (2002) Policy Position Paper on Capacity and Consent. Age Concern England Policy Unit, London.

Age Concern Institute of Gerontology, Centre of Medical Law and Ethics (1988) *The Living Will: consent to treatment at the end of life, a Working Party report*. Edward Arnold, London.

American Bar Association. www.abanet.org.

British Medical Association (1995) *Advance Statements About Medical Treatment: Code of Practice with explanatory notes*. BMA, London.

Costello, J. (2000) *Law and Finance in Retirement*. Blackhall, Dublin.

Dickens, B. (1993) 'A response to the papers of Molloy and colleagues (Canada) and Cranford (United States) on advance directives.' *Humane Medicine*, 9 (1): 80.

Docker, C. (1996) 'Advance directives/Living Wills.' In McLean, S. (ed.) *Contemporary Issues in Law, Medicine and Ethics*. Dartmouth Publishing, Aldershot.

Emmanuel, E., Emmanuel, L. (1992) 'Four models of the physician–patient relationship.' *Journal of the American Medical Association*, 267 (16): 2221–2225.

Emanuel, L., Emanuel, E. (1993) 'Decisions at the end of life communicated by patients.' *Hastings Center Report*, Sept–Oct: 6.

High, D. (1993) 'Advance directives and the elderly.' *Gerontologist*, 33 (3): 347.

Holt, J. 'Withdrawing treatment: ethical issues at the end of life', in Kendrick, K., Clarke, D. and Flanagan, J. (2002) *Advancing Nursing Practice in Cancer Care Ethics*. Palgrave, Basingstoke.

Irvine of Lairg (1999) *Mental Incapacity – New Millennium, New Law?* Speech to the Law Society Conference on Mental Incapacity, 10 November, London. Also available on www.lcd.gov.uk/speeches/1999/1999.htm).

Jeffrey, P. (2001) *Going Against the Stream: ethical aspects of ageing and care*. Gracewing, Leominster.

Kutner, L. (1969) 'Due process of euthanasia: the Living Will, a proposal.' *Indiana Law Review*, 44: 539–554.

La Puma, J., Orentlichner, D., Moss, R. (1991) 'Advance directives on admission.' *Journal of the American Medical Association*, 266 (3): 402–405.

Law Commission (1995) *Mental Incapacity Report 231*. HMSO, London.

Lord Chancellor's Department (1997) *Who Decides? Making decisions on behalf of mentally incapacitated adults*. HMSO, London.

Lord Chancellor's Office (1999) *Making Decisions: the Government's proposals for making decisions on behalf of mentally incapacitated adults (Cm 4465)*. The Stationery Office, London.

Luttrell, S., Sommerville, A. (1996) 'Limiting risks by curtailing rights: a response to Dr Ryan.' *Journal of Medical Ethics*, 27 (3): 274–277.

McHale, J. (1998) 'Mental incapacity: some proposals for legislative reform.' *Journal of Medical Ethics*, 24: 322–327.

McHale, J., Fox, M. (1997) *Health Care Law*. Sweet and Maxwell, London.

Montgomery, J. (1994) 'Power over death: the final sting.' In Lee, R., Morgan, D. (eds.) *Death Rites: law and ethics at the end of life*. Routledge, London.

Molloy, D.W., Mepham, V. (1990) *Let Me Decide*, 2e. McMaster University Press, Ontario.

Patients' Association (1996) *Advance Statements About Future Medical Treatment*. The Patients' Association, London.

Sam, M., Singer, P. (1993) 'Canadian outpatients and advance directives.' *Canadian Medical Association Journal*, 148 (9): 1497–1502.

Scottish Executive (1999) *Making the Right Moves: rights and protection for adults with incapacity (SE/1999/24)*. Scottish Office, Edinburgh.

Seckler, A. (1991) 'Substituted judgement: how accurate are proxy predictions?' *Annals of Internal Medicine*, 117: 599–606.

Silva, M.C., Sorrell, J.M. (1984) 'Factors influencing comprehension of information for informed consent; ethical implications for nursing research.' *International Journal of Nursing Studies*, 21 (4): 233–240.

Society for the Protection of the Unborn Child (1998) *Beyond Autonomy. Response to the Green Paper, 'Who Decides?'* SPUC, London.

Sommerville, A. (1996) 'Are advance directives really the answer? And what was the question?' In McLean, S. (ed.) *Death, Dying and the Law*. Dartmouth Publishing, Aldershot.

United States Living Will Registry. www.uslivingwillregistry.com/fedregs.shtm

Wilson, L. (1999) *Living Wills*. Nursing Times Monographs, London.

4 The Ethical Debate

Core moral themes

Underlying the legal debates of the last chapter, especially concerning common law, are the basic ethical principles which have to be addressed in order to reach a balanced and fair decision. In this chapter we will look at the ethical themes underlying the legal debate. Our aim is not to argue for a particular ethical position but rather to review the debate, clarify the ethical issues and examine the implications for the health care practitioner.

We will focus on the six major areas of ethical reflection in advance directives:

- The principle of *autonomy*
- The issue of *futile treatment*
- The question of *identity*
- *Respect* for human life
- Advance directives for *research*
- The nature of *ethical decision making* in this context. This includes practical questions as to exactly what difference an advance directive might actually make.

Autonomy

As we saw in the last chapter, the principle of autonomy – self rule – is the basic moral ground for advance statements. Autonomy involves 'mastery of self, the ability to decide for oneself, balancing competing views' (Wilson 1999:7). The moral argument goes back to the issue of consent. Patients have to have control over their body, and thus have the right to refuse treatment, the right to self-determination. In advance directives this same right is simply extended to a time when the person is no longer able to direct the treatment.

Critics of this principle argue that the underlying view of autonomy is not adequate, based as it seems to be on a liberal philosophical view.

Four arguments range against this view of autonomy:

- That it is individualistic
- That it denies social justice
- That it cannot accept any form of paternalism
- That it ignores the importance of personal relationships.

Individualism

The liberal view of autonomy is based on an individualist view of the self. This sees the self as 'atomistic', and 'independent', set apart from the network of relationships which form community. Hence, the important underlying freedom is one of choice and control. This forms the basis of Berlin's *negative freedom*, freedom from the oppression or the control of the other (Berlin 1969). This leads to arguments that focus on the threat of paternalism, and interference with the choice of the patient.

Against this is the communitarian view of the person that sees him or her as located in community, not independent of or prior to it (McIntyre 1981, Sandel 1984). Thus, the person cannot be seen in an atomistic, dislocated way but rather finds identity, convictions and purpose from the community in which he or she exists.

In fact, such a debate sets up a false dichotomy between freedom and community, one which mischaracterises the modern view of liberalism and also the nature of community. As Ikonomidis and Singer (1999) note, modern liberalism is concerned not so much with an individual's independence and choice, but rather with that individual's ownership of and responsibility for personal values, the decision making process, and thus character itself. Hence, 'a person is autonomous when he or she understands the development of and changes in his or her character' (Ikonomidis and Singer 1999:523). Such a judgement of, and responsibility for, the self can only take place in the light of our social and historical context. Thus, modern liberals recognise that it is impossible to think of ourselves except as 'part of ongoing communities, defined by reciprocal bonds of obligation, common traditions and institutions' (Ikonomidis and Singer 1999:523). What the liberal objects to is the possibility of the individuality and uniqueness of a person being swallowed up by the collective mass.

On the other side the view that the community provides the significant narrative, which gives meaning and purpose to the person, cannot stand by itself. Few communities have one simple narrative providing meaning for all members. Even religious communities, such as the Christian church, tend to encompass very different perspectives. Moreover, most people are members of several different communities and develop their meaning not so much in the light of single narrative but rather in the light of the dialogue between the very different narratives in their lives (Robinson 2001, Chapter 3). This is the essence of what is often referred to as 'post-modernism'. Moral meaning is not summed up in one major ethical narrative. On the contrary there are many different, often local, narratives and any broader understanding demands dialogue between the different narrative, affirming similarities and living with difference (Bauman 1993). In the light of this, individuality and with that moral autonomy, emerges from the capacity to engage in such dialogue.

Denial of social justice

A second objection to the liberal view of autonomy is that it entails the denial of social justice. The critics argue that the stress on the rights of individuals to determine their own treatment through advance directives is a form of consumerism, with individual choice being given more weight than the concerns and needs of society at large (Childress and Fletcher 1994). Once again, however, this is to hold a mistaken view of liberal autonomy. Ikonomidis and Singer (1999: 524) argue that as a practical matter advance directives which request certain treatment can be overridden in the light of broader principles and issues to do with the just distribution of health care.

Hence, the proper liberal view of autonomy in advance care planning is not about guaranteeing whatever the patient wants, but rather 'the responsible use of freedom'. The right course of action in this light may not be one that promotes the interest of the individual but of the family as a whole. In this socially responsible approach to advance directives 'the patient is viewed as both citizen and consumer, and patient self determination is viewed in the context of "informed consent" rather than in the context of "consumer sovereignty"'(Ikonomidis and Singer 1999:524). Modern liberalism then is not simply concerned with the protection of rights and liberties, but rather the protection of such liberties in the context of good decision making which takes into account the needs of others and an underlying egalitarian conception of justice.

Unjustifiable paternalism

A third objection to so called liberal autonomy is that it cannot accept any paternalism as justifiable. This is especially difficult for advance directives since the whole principle of substituted judgement involves a degree of paternalism in trying to determine the scope of the directive and in ensuring that best interest of the patient is taken into account.

However, modern liberalism is not dead set against the idea of paternalism *per se*. It is concerned that respect for the right to self-determination be recognised, but notes certain situations in which paternalism is acceptable. Ikonomidis and Singer (1999) call attention to the modern liberal distinction between 'hard paternalism' and 'soft paternalism'. The first imposes values and judgements on people 'for their own good', something opposed by liberalism. This paternalism is something that the medical world has been systemically guilty of in the past. The doctor has been seen as having power over the patient and as knowing what is best for the patient (Campbell 1984). Soft paternalism, however, accepts the right of the state to prevent self-regarding harm when conduct is non-voluntary, that is to say where the consent is missing. This protects the autonomous person against possible external coercion. In respect of advance directives it is also important, for instance, in making decisions for the patient about treatments that may not have been known about or understood by the patient when the directive was made. This allows such interference based upon the best interest principle. Hence, liberalism is able to justify basic paternalistic restrictions, provided that they do not run counter to directives which have fulfilled the legal and moral criteria, including decisions arrived at without any coercion.

A great deal of the debate about autonomy once more involves a simplistic opposing of paternalism and liberalism. Moreover, this often characterises the medical establishment as a whole as paternalistic.

While this has been true of the establishment in the past there are increasing examples of the medical profession breaking away from such attitudes and enabling patients to participate in their own treatment and choice of treatment (BMA 1995). The debate points to the need for frameworks and procedures which will both guard against the abuse of hard paternalism and ensure that decision making respects and involves patients and all relevant persons.

It is worth noting that some writers do argue for a more hard-line paternalism. Shimon Glick, for instance, argues for the morality of coercion (Glick 2000). This is based upon the Israeli Patients' Rights Law (1996) which permits coercing a competent patient into accepting life-saving therapy 'if an ethics committee feels that if treatment is imposed the patient will give his/her consent retroactively' (p. 393).

Ignoring the importance of personal relationships

The fourth objection to a liberal view of autonomy is that it does not account for the importance of personal relationships. This is a development of the first objection. Often set out by feminist ethicists it argues that the liberal view of autonomy is atomistic and above all does not take account of the inherently social nature of human being and of the 'relatedness' which precedes and is a condition of autonomy (Nedelsky 1989). Feminist writers argue further that the concern for principles, justice and protection from coercion is not the right basis for a medical ethic. They suggest more an ethic of care and 'connectedness' that would ensure that all parties were involved in decision making (Koehn 1998).

Ikonomidis and Singer (1999) accept that the liberal position does not spend much time on the nature and value of personal relationships and how these might affect decision making. Nonetheless, they argue (p. 526) that liberalism is 'not inconsistent with an account of the nature and value of personal relationships in health care planning'. Modern liberalism therefore should be developed in terms of preserving and protecting such relationships.

The debate on liberal autonomy versus paternalism, then, provides two important conclusions. Firstly, the polarisation of autonomy and paternalism is wrongly characterised. Far from being either/or, there should be concern for both the freedom of the individual, and for the community in which that individual develops personal values and makes decisions. Secondly, this wider ethical debate leads the modern liberal to supplement the need to protect, with concern for personal relationships. As a result, the advance directive has to be seen in the light of the patient's network of relationships.

This ethical debate and the need for balance is reflected in the legal developments. Firstly, there is stress on the need for consent to treatment as the baseline protection against any coercive paternalism. Secondly, there is reluctance to make directives legally binding. The stress is rather on dialogue and relationships. Thirdly, the Government's concern for the use of attorneys and managers provides a framework that aims to balance all of these factors.

This move away from a simplistic view is also reflected in research which points to a more profound view of advance planning from patients themselves.

In one qualitative study of 48 patients receiving haemodialysis the view of the patients involved four significant elements:

- The purpose of advance planning was not simply preparing for incapacity but preparing for death
- The central issues of advance care planning were not simply about the wishes of the patient but concern for others, not least in relieving possible burdens
- The focus for advance planning should not be simply the written form but also the social decision making process
- The context of advance planning has to be the family and friends as much as the physician/ patient relationship (Singer *et al.* 1998).

Such findings have been subsequently confirmed in other research, on such topics as concern about preparing for death, achieving a sense of control, and the strengthening of significant relationships (Martin *et al.* 1999). Concerns of this nature take us beyond simple ethical matters into areas of personal worth and ultimate meaning, areas variously described as existential or spiritual. This in turn takes the focus, even for modern liberals, away from the simplistic view of autonomy to the concept of shared governance, which recognises that effective decision making is not possible without collaboration in aspects such as data gathering, and putting into practice preferred options (Marriner-Tomey 1993). This will be examined more closely in the final section below.

Futile treatment

An important part of the debate about patient autonomy and the advance directive has been the question of defining medical futility. As Halliday puts it this is not simply an abstract argument, 'but is part of a three way struggle for control within and around the practice of medicine' (Halliday 1997). He notes one American survey in 1995 which found that 96 per cent of doctors had withheld or withdrawn life support treatment on the expectation of the patient's death, sometimes without the knowledge or consent of the patient or the patient's surrogate (Asch *et al.* 1995). Behind this is an assumption of power, and of the proper role of the doctor to make decisions. Hence, the BMA report of 1988 advocated respect for advance statements but refused to see them as binding:

> 'At times a judicious medical paternalism may well be the best and most realistic way to achieve a good outcome where the situation is not quite as the declarer might have envisaged it.' (Quoted in Greaves 1989:182)

This approach has been heavily criticised, with one commentator going so far as to suggest that 'futility' was being used as a 'crowbar' to take 'a certain type of decision making away from the patients to the physicians' (Nelson 1994). Taking an opposing view, writers such as Paris and Reardon have argued that this can lead to negative effects, not least the reduction of the doctor as a moral agent who has professional responsibilities for assessing and enabling good decisions. They can become transformed into 'mere extensions of the patient's whim, fantasy, or unrealistic hopes and desires' (Paris and Reardon 1992).

The third part of the power struggle has been the medical insurance companies in the USA and the National Health Service in the UK. By definition they are trying to control costs and determine what is proper care coverage (Halliday 1997:149).

Clearly an agreed definition of futile treatment would break down this struggle, providing freedom for the doctor from having to provide medical treatment and freedom for the state in providing resources.

At the heart of this has been debate about the very concept of futility. Several definitions of futile procedures have been offered, including:

- 'Failing to prolong life' (Brett and McCullough 1986)
- 'Failing to achieve the patient's wishes' (Blackhall 1987)
- 'Failing to achieve a therapeutic benefit for the patient' (Youngner 1988).

Schneiderman and Jecker define a futile action as one 'that cannot achieve the goals of the action, no matter how often repeated' (1993). The hope was that a purely physiological definition could be arrived at, that is one that would be value neutral. However, as Halliday argues, it is hard, if not impossible, to establish such a definition. At one level it is hard to find conclusive evidence for a simple physiological view of futility (Halliday 1997). More importantly Schneiderman, Faber-Langendoen and Jecker (1994) argue that this view of futility focuses purely on the medical model of health, 'a reductionist approach that is incompatible with medicine, placing primary values on organ function and body substance'. They argue that this approach is itself a 'value choice' which moves away from the person centred approach to medicine.

In addition, Halliday argues that any idea of futility must take into account the benefit not only to the individual person, but also to the wider constituency. Loewy and Carlson (1993) give the instance of a situation where treatment would be futile for the patient but where it is important to maintain some treatment in order to allow the family to come to terms with the death of the person and be involved in the process.

Another argument against the attempt to use futility as the single criterion is the danger of not taking into account other possible principles, not least the sanctity of human life, as if they had no relevance (Halliday 1997).

So, while it is important to have some definition of physiological futility, this has to be seen within in a social context including an acceptable account of the relationships between patient, doctor and family members, and with reference to a broader set of values and principles. Hence, advance directives cannot hope to rely purely upon an agreed definition of futility, but have to be worked out in the context of the various relationships.

Identity

As we saw in Case Study 3.1, in the previous chapter, many questions can be raised about the identity of the person who may be incapacitated. Before suffering dementia, John was a lively person who gloried in the academic exchange. His very sense of identity and worth was based on the capacity to achieve this. After developing the dementia, however, John was 'no longer himself'. He became utterly dependent, and had no means of self-determination. Moreover, he lost the capacity that was central to his life. But his second son Geoff saw something positive in this change. He felt his father had actually begun to find part of his more holistic self, expressing feelings through body language and touch. Geoff would sit for hours holding his father's hand and all the while John was neither distressed nor in pain. The holding, moreover, was not merely a passive activity. At times John would push hard against his son's hand. At other times he would hug him or explore his face with his fingers. John appeared to live a happy life simply looking at flowers in the garden and taking tea, a life where he accepted the care of others and did not need to achieve. In a real sense John was at peace with himself. Should life-saving treatment be withheld on the basis of what seems to be quite another person's view?

Dworkin (1993) accepts the complexity of such situations and argues that in dementia there appear to be two different persons. He writes of two autonomies as being in play – that of the demented patient and of the person who became demented. This duality can lead to potential conflict. Nonetheless, it is not possible to say that the person has changed their mind. On the contrary it is simply that this person is no longer able to frame or express their values. Dworkin then argues that there are certain 'critical values' which give purpose, coherence and meaning to our lives, and these should take precedence. An individual's life is more than simply the different moments that make it up, it has to be seen as whole. In this light, the integrity of the person and the consistency of their life meaning must be respected. The advance directive provides this consistency, giving voice to the critical values. Olick echoes many of these points arguing that the law often seems to treat persons newly judged as incompetent as devoid of their past. Such a past is still part of the narrative which informs the person's present identity and situation (Olick 2001).

Tony Hope (1996) argues against this on two grounds:

1 The person who makes a directive against life saving treatment in the context of dementia assumes that this must be an experience that would be at best without awareness and at worse involving either emotional pain or a loss of dignity. The person would in all probability have failed to imagine the possibility of a state of being such as that apparently experienced by John, where he seemed satisfied and happy.
2 The case of dementia must be distinguished from a simple coma. The person with dementia is still able to feel experiences which may give pleasure or pain. More adventurously, Hope argues that a person's values can be communicated not only through explicitly cognitive communication but also through affective and somatic ways, such as body language and touch. How we treat such a person then 'should not be determined by his former wishes, based on different values which are no longer of relevance to him' (Hope 1996, 68).

Hope then suggests another example to test Dworkin's thesis. In this he assumes a man who, rather than valuing the intellect, values an individualistic machismo approach to life. He may pride himself on not having anaesthetic at the dentist and state in his advance directive that he should have no painkillers or sedatives. Should this directive then be followed when the same person becomes demented and is suffering severe toothache? The person is not competent to balance the concern for his pain against his 'critical interest'. Indeed, it could be said that in that case the critical interest only really applies when the patient is aware. It is the very nature of the individualistic machismo effort against suffering that the person should be fully aware.

Underlying this are two factors. Firstly, the desire of the competent person may well go against or compete with the wellbeing of the person who is demented. Secondly, and connected, the desire of the competent person may be based upon values which are at the least contestable. In this case the expressed values of the person are based upon an individualism which has to prove itself through suffering and which cannot accept any dependency upon another. This in turn views dignity purely in terms of independence. However, in the experience of dementia there may be a simple acceptance of others, which may represent an equally valid view of dignity. This must not be romanticised; caring for demented persons who are doubly incontinent is not easy.

Christopher Ryan takes the argument further, albeit focusing on cases where the condition of incompetence is potentially reversible, and examines the underlying psychology of advance directives. Critically, he argues that 'Human beings ... are very poor at determining their attitudes to treatment for some hypothetical future terminal illness and very frequently grossly underestimate their future desire to go on living' (Ryan 1996:96). Ryan accounts for this theoretically through the idea of denial. In effect he argues that the person denies the possibility of a difficult death through opting for a hypothetical early death. This, however, is precisely an unrealistic view of death and dying. Indeed, he argues, one can only begin to understand what it means to die when faced with the possibility. At that point most people look to survival.

Hope (1996) describes one patient who suffered a stroke from which she eventually recovered. Her advance directive said that during major illness such as a stroke she should not be given active treatment. Still aware during the illness, she was above all concerned to live and was intensely anxious about the possibility of her doctors following her advance directive. In her case, she had to rely upon the judgement of the doctors.

Ryan also notes a number of relevant studies in psychiatric literature which suggest preference for intervention in an episode of serious illness. One study examined the ability of future treatment choices and discovered that in cases where patients had been into hospital, or suffered accidents, the choices tended to change with more intervention being preferred in future treatment. Another found that in patients with cancer those with good prognosis had the strongest interest in euthanasia while those with the poorer prognosis, offered only palliative treatment, tended to reject euthanasia as a possible option (Ryan 1996:96).

Based on this, Ryan maintains the autonomy argument for the advance directive is no longer relevant. In a real sense, individuals cannot truly know what it is to be faced with the scenario about which they are hypothesising. The patient 'does not know that it is highly likely that her decision, made now, that she would rather die if faced with a hypothetical future scenario is not what her decision would have been were she actually faced with that scenario'.

Ryan's argument has its problems. Taken to extremes it would make it impossible for anyone to plan for anything, simply because they have never experienced or been faced with that thing. As Luttrell and Sommerville (1996) also note, there is every reason to believe that if individuals were to make their advance directive in close dialogue with medical staff and family, then they could form a good idea of what the experience might be like. In any case Ryan does seem to underestimate the capacity of persons to face up to the possibility of future suffering or death.

Nonetheless, the experience of a life-threatening situation is not an everyday one, and this whole section of the debate raises major questions about reliance on an advance directive form which might deny the autonomy of the incapacitated patient, as much as it might celebrate it. An example of this was raised by Rosner (1994) in a *Lancet* article. An elderly woman had advanced cancer of the colon and intestinal obstruction. The pain was not amenable to painkillers, but could have been relieved by a colostomy under local anaesthetic. Her advance directive, however, forbade any 'heroic' intervention in the case of incurable illness and did not differentiate between treatment that would prolong life or relieve pain. Such a case highlights the impossibility of simply favouring one view of autonomy and supports the view that any directive has to be part of an overall process. The Government's conclusions, with their baseline of concern for self-determination and overview of best interest, are an attempt to ensure this balance. Under present guidelines it would have been possible to provide the operation precisely because the advance directive did not foresee this kind of dilemma.

Some writers, such as Sommerville (1996) and Kutner (1969), propose a way out of the identity problem through simply treating the body as a possession. Kutner's original idea was about an advance document 'analogous to a revocable or conditional trust, with the patient's body as *res* (the property or asset), the patient as the beneficiary and grantor, and the doctor and hospital as trustees' (Kutner 1969). The problem with this approach is that in the case of dementia it would categorise the living body as *res*, when in fact it is precisely the personhood of the demented patient which is being argued by Ryan (1996) and Hope (1996). Their argument, however, has problems when applied to forms of dementia which are likened to persistent vegetative state (Pallis and Harley 1995).

The debate about identity then does not give a knock down resolution to the advance directive issue. Instead it once more focuses us on the social networks and underlying life meaning which form the basis of any ethical and pastoral judgement.

Respect for life; respect for God

Respect for human life can be taken to be the irreducible moral attitude. Since the Holocaust this has been reinforced through the work of writers such as Zygmunt Bauman (Bauman 1993).

Underlying respect for human life has been a long tradition of natural law. Natural law is associated with religious ethics, though not exclusively so. It argues that an ethical judgement should be based upon the natural law, which is arrived at through rational reflection on the *telos*, or purpose of any created thing. Hence, for example, if the purpose of marriage is primarily procreation then whatever prevents that purpose is wrong. Natural law sees certain principles as fundamental, in particular respect for human life, leading to the moral principle that it is wrong to take life. Often associated with this in theological terms is the principle of the sovereignty of God, the belief that we should not take away from God what is rightfully His task, giving and taking of life. Both of these can be used in relation to the advance directive argument, not least where the refusal to give consent might lead to death.

Sovereignty of God

This argument can be misleading and confusing in that it could be used for or against advance directives. The use of medical technology is precisely something that can prevent the natural course of the person's life. Hence, to ensure that it is not used in certain situations might be proper. On the other hand to withdraw treatment might be said to take things into ones own hands – taking away from God's task.

The sovereignty of God argument raises major theological problems for whichever faith uses it. If God is sovereign in the sense of Him not simply creating the world but also controlling the death of each person, we have to ask why some die and others do not. Most importantly it raises the question of why some die 'early' or 'less well'. Even more problematic is the idea of what might be a natural end to life. Taken to its logical end this would lead to the conclusion that no medical intervention is proper, thus putting into question all the improvements in medical care which have led, for instance, to increased life expectancy and improvements in the quality of life (Badham 1998). From a different perspective medical intervention could be seen as working with God's plans. Such a collaborative view is equally possible.

Most faiths share a view of God's sovereignty. Islam argues that the person is not absolute owner of his or her life. Moreover, where life is taken away this affects post mortem relationships with God. Moreover, like some Christian and Buddhist strands they hold a positive view of human suffering, as enabling spiritual growth (Morgan and Lawton 1996:247). Hindu writers stress that there is a right time (*kala*) for death. At the same time they hold a view of the acceptability of the *willed death*, where a man may control his dying by refusing to take any food or drink (Morgan and Lawton 1996:33).

Respect for human life

Although this is not exclusively a religious principle, it is often articulated by the Christian churches. Pope John Paul notes that the basis of such respect is that man is created in the image of God (*Genesis* 1:26–28), and that the dignity which this gives to human beings is inviolable. The principle of human dignity is of course shared by other faiths, including Judaism, Buddhism, Hinduism and Islam (see Armstrong, Dixon and Robinson 1999: 12–13). The Pope continues:

'If such great care must be taken to respect every life, even that of criminals and unjust aggressors, the commandment, "You shall not kill", has absolute value when it refers to the innocent person. And all the more so in the case of the weak defenceless human being … In effect, the absolute inviolability of innocent human life is a moral truth, clearly taught by Sacred Scriptures, constantly upheld in the Church's tradition and consistently proposed by her Magisterium.' (John Paul II 1995, 57, paragraphs 1 and 2)

Based on this, the Pope argues that euthanasia is morally unacceptable. This forms the bottom line in judging the advance directive. As Archbishop Yong of Singapore notes, the church recognises the right of self-determination in medical decisions, including the refusal of life-sustaining treatment (Yong 1995). In the situation where a person is dying, the refusal of treatment which would extend life unreasonably is acceptable in terms of natural law. Hence, the Pope distinguishes euthanasia from the decision to forego 'aggressive medical treatment', ie 'medical procedures which no longer correspond to the real situation of the patient, either because they are by now disproportionate to any expected results or because they impose an excessive burden on the patient and his family' (quoted in Yong 1995: 2). In such situations, where death is imminent and inevitable, Pope John Paul argues that it is possible 'to refuse forms of treatment that would only secure a precarious and burdensome prolongation of life, so long as the normal care due to a sick person in such circumstances is not interrupted'. All of this is not the equivalent of suicide or euthanasia, but rather expresses 'acceptance of the human condition in the face of death' (Yong 1995).

Yong explores the connection between euthanasia and the advance directive. While he does not oppose the advance directive as such, he is very aware of a strong connection with euthanasia. Even though no intrinsic connection is spelt out, he does see the potential for a 'slippery slope'. As the idea takes hold so it raises the danger of desensitising all involved to the connection between advance directives and the death of the patient. The difference between not wanting treatment and wanting to die becomes obscured. Because of this possibility, Yong argues that it is important not to enshrine advance directives in legislation. Moreover, the necessary consultation between medical staff and family is already there and encouraged, and the principles of common law do not demand doctors maintain futile treatment. He argues that, in any case, legislation for advance directives has achieved little, rather making the issues more complex. Peter Jeffrey supports this argument, and points to further complexity (Jeffrey 2001:99–100). It is always assumed that the refusal of treatment will lead to the end of life. However, there remains a chance in any situation that the patient will not die, thus remaining bed-bound for a significant time, in possibly an even worse situation than was feared.

The Society for the Protection of Unborn Children (SPUC) takes such arguments further in its response to the Green paper *'Who Decides?'* (SPUC 1998). The Society was particularly concerned that under possible future legislation, and even under common law, the advance directive could become a means of assisted suicide or euthanasia. In support of this view, it quotes an advance directive drawn up by the Voluntary Euthanasia Society:

'I wish it to be understood that I fear degeneration and indignity far more than I fear death. I ask my medical attendant to bear this in mind when considering what my intention would be in any uncertain situation'.

SPUC argues that this is likely to be seen as 'indication to the contrary', which overrides presumption in favour of life saving treatment. It is likely, that a statement so worded, especially when made by a member of the Voluntary Euthanasia Society, is based on a belief that life loses its value under certain conditions and that its end is not merely tolerable but may become the object of one's intentions' (SPUC 1998:9).

In these circumstances, if the advance directive is binding once the patient is incapacitated, it becomes an instrument of the author's intention to cause his or her own death. While this would be legally acceptable, because there is no explicit direction involving the death of the patient, SPUC argues that it would be morally unacceptable.

This creates very murky water indeed, including the possibility of the patient trying actively to deceive the medical staff into action that would lead to death. Most parties are clear that there is a real distinction between allowing death to take its natural course and actually taking life (Kennedy 1997). However, if advance directives were to be binding, regardless of the situation, there would be a danger of obscuring that distinction. Fear of misuse then begins to chip away at the respect for human life, and the trust on which such respect is based.

HOPE (Healthcare Opposed to Euthanasia) goes further to challenge the view that tube feeding is not always intrusive care, and from this argues that withdrawal of this can be intentional killing:

> 'Recognising that a majority see tube feeding in cases of persistent vegetative state as futile treatment in someone who is effectively dead already, we, however, are convinced that tube feeding can be an effective part of the basic care all living beings deserve simply because they are human and living. To withdraw it in the case of PVS is the intentional killing by omission of someone who is not dying in any previously understood sense of that word.' (HOPE 1998)

Against this it could be argued the point about persistent vegetative state (PVS) is precisely that it does not fit into any simple category. Far from not fitting into a process of dying, it is in itself a form of death. Where there is no hope of recovery it is a state that can be deemed to be unacceptable, and thus the withdrawal of tube feeding cannot be viewed as killing.

The recent cases of Diane Pretty and 'Miss B' exemplify some of the ethical issues that begin to surface. For many they point to a clear distinction between assisted suicide and euthanasia, and refusal of treatment. Diane Pretty lost her case to the European Court of Human Rights to make her husband immune from prosecution should he assist her suicide (BMA news briefing, 29 April, 2002). 'Miss B' was a tetraplegic on a ventilator. She won her case to refuse this treatment, having been found to be competent to make this decision (*BMJ* 2002, 324:629). Miss B's case was a simple example of negative freedom, preventing someone from imposing a treatment that was not acceptable to the person. Though the outcome would have been the same, the case of Diane Pretty goes beyond that of Miss B, involving an active taking of life and setting this up as a human right. Against this, Baroness Warnock argues that there is no real distinction between so called 'active' killing and withdrawal of treatment. She derides the underlying mythology:

> 'It is as if to cause someone's death, death it is necessary to hit or stab or shoot or inject with poison. But, as common sense tells us, I can kill my cat by neglecting to feed it as well as by shooting it, though the death may be longer.' (Warnock 2002)

However, whilst Mary Warnock's comparison makes reasonable sense, it can hardly be applied directly to a situation where treatment which might lead to death is consciously withdrawn. Nor does it begin to answer the underlying feelings of many in the medical profession who find even the withdrawal of treatment to be a difficult option. Warnock's debate inevitably leads on to the question of how a decision is made, which both respects the law as it stands and also involves all concerned more fully. This will be developed below.

As a response to the debate on refusal of treatment in general, the General Medical Council are, at the time of writing, about to issue guidelines on good practice in decision making for withholding and withdrawing life-prolonging treatments (www.gmc-uk.org). This sets out standards of practice expected of doctors in this area, and follows broadly the advice of the BMA.

In the meantime the basic idea of respect for life remains important. It forms the basis of the arguments from both HOPE and SPUC that the non-competent patient who has not given advance communication should be carefully protected. However, its greatest problem is its generality. What it means in any situation is not clear. It could be argued that respect for human life is not simply about keeping patients alive but about the quality of that life. Hence, those who argue for refusal will tend to use this principle in their favour. It can equally be used to argue against non use or withdrawal of treatment (Kennedy and Grubb 1994:1197).

Advance directives, research and resources

Up to this point patient autonomy and life choice have been the key reasons for advance directives. It is possible to see other, altruistic reasons, including permitting research on patients with dementia, and the use of advance directives to manage limited resources.

The first of these, advance directives for non-therapeutic dementia research, is criticised by Berghams (1998) on moral and practical grounds. He argues with Parfit, against Dworkin, that the personal identity is not the same throughout life. There are different stages in life where the person may hold very different views based on different spiritual and ethical perspectives, such that it is not possible to make decisions for the future person (Parfit 1979). Perhaps more critically there is the danger of the demented person being used simply as a research object. One of the key definitions of respect for persons is it does not involve using the other for our ends, however laudable they may be. The personhood of the demented person must always be assumed.

A different view, from John Harris (1985), suggests that the fundamental criterion for personhood is the individual's capacity to assess and value their life. The problem with this argument is its exclusivity. It takes away the value of personhood from a whole range of individuals, from children to people with a learning disability. Reflecting upon the Holocaust, Bauman argues that the fundamental ethical stance is to assume the personhood of the 'other'. Without this there is always the danger of the slippery slope and the definition and redefinition of categories of human beings who do not befit the term 'person' (Bauman 1993).

Practical objections include recruitment for research. Few advance directives are made for such research and given the difficulty of finding a healthy patient who would fill this in, then dementing patients will have to be consulted in the early stages of their illness. However, many symptoms go undetected until a severe stage has been reached (Berghams 1998:35).

Perhaps most crucially, if research were the main aim of the doctor who was advising advance directives it is possible that this would affect trust in that doctor. There is the danger of seeing concern for some other thing not the patient. A similar argument exists against the use of advance directives for saving costs on treatment. As we saw above this might be seen as way of helping to steward limited resources. However, if this were seen as a possible motive then it would create suspicion and mistrust in any doctor who encouraged the making of an advance directive (Sommerville 1996:43).

Nonetheless, it is possible to see the development of advance directives which authorise rather than refuse treatment that could have positive good for the patient and for others. A patient who already carries a donor card, for instance, might agree to elective ventilation for organ harvesting. Or a mother facing incapacity might agree in advance to genetic testing which she does not herself need but which may benefit her offspring. The Government is encouraging the more positive use of advance directives and, as Sommerville (1996) notes, the development of advance directives historically has been from refusal to positive treatment.

Such creative use of the advance directive once more focuses on the need to get right the decision making process, so that patients can reflect on the full range of options which are most relevant to them, and thus maximise the creativity. Hence, we must now turn to a more detailed examination of the decision making process.

The ethical decision making process

The principle of best interest has been seen by some as a classic example of the paternalistic approach of the medical profession. In the end the judgement about what will happen comes down to the professional. Thus the autonomy of the patient is once more compromised, so the argument goes (Wilson 1999).

Ardagh (1999), however, suggests that the principles underlying this and the idea of professional substituted judgement are far from paternalistic. He calls on the four fundamental principles set out by Beauchamp and Childress (2001) for decision making in medical ethics:

- Respect
- Beneficence
- Non-maleficence
- Justice.

Analysis of these different principles reveals that they force the doctor to move beyond any simple paternalistic stance. Firstly, **respect** involves respect for the autonomy of the patient. Basically this means treating the patient as a person, a subject who can make decisions. In the case of the person who is not competent, the doctor must find out the thoughts and feelings of the patient.

The principle of **beneficence** involves the concern for the best outcome for the patient. This is very much the principle of best interest. Once again this cannot be discovered from any pre-set idea or principle. What is best for the patient can only be seen in dialogue with patient. Like the question of futility, best interest is not simply a physiological question.

The principle of **non-maleficence** looks to the avoidance of harm. In assessing whether invasive treatment should be applied the harm that this may cause has to be taken into account. Once again the final understanding of harm is not simply physiological and can only be worked out in relation to the particular case.

Justice is about the attempt to respect all equally and provide equal treatment. This, of course, is never actually possible. Hence, justice tends to be about providing the treatment that is appropriate for the person. Above all it involves not excluding people from treatment on grounds other than need.

All four principles have in practice to be held in balance and in turn inform the instrumental principles which begin to enable the more general principles to be put into practice. Beauchamp and Childress (2001) note four instrumental principles:

- **Confidentiality.** This is an expression of the respect for the person. Information which is particular to the patient and which might be embarrassing is not shared. The sensibilities of the patient are attended to.

- **Informed consent.** Informed consent enables the person to develop a genuinely autonomous capacity. The positive view of autonomy is one which sees the person developing an awareness. Most importantly the logic of informed consent is that the doctor presents the patient with diagnosis and the proposed treatment, with estimates of success, and enables the patient to make a decision. This is not a straightforward process, even for a competent person who has to decide about treatment in the present. It may involve working through emotional difficulties in both accepting the diagnosis and also in working through implications of the treatment. It is even more difficult for the patient who is not competent, as we have seen, not least in knowing if the directive actually applies to this situation.
- **Cost–benefit analysis and Risk–benefit analysis**. Both of these enable beneficence and non-maleficence to be worked through, in the light of constraints and resources. How far will the available resources enable the benefit of the patient to be worked through? What are the risks to the patient and what are the constraints to avoiding those risks? They have often been criticised in the past and yet they are central in any attempt to work through a decision, seen purely as a form of utilitarian calculus. However, constraints to delivery of care cannot be ignored and in any case risk and cost are not seen simply in financial or physiological terms but involve broader questions, such as dignity and human relationships which the doctor ought to be aware of. The key point is that these are instrumental principles that should be seen as enabling the major principles to be affected.

The stages of decision making

The decision making process involves:

- Data gathering
- Value clarification
- Negotiation of responsibility
- Estimate of options in the light of resources and constraints.

Several things stand out in this process:

1 At no point is decision making simply individualistic. In all these stages there needs to be collaboration. Ardagh (1999) argues that the doctor in the case of emergency has to make the decision based upon professional substituted judgement. Even this needs others to help bring the data about the person to life. This means either the advance directive or the proxy.

2 Value clarification leads beyond the simple uncritical acceptance of principles. It takes the patient on to examine values in relation to her life and the different relationships (Robinson 2001). For many people this is a reflective process they have never been through and one which is only brought to the fore when faced by a crisis or the possibility of crisis. Such values have an affective and cognitive dimension and often need another present to enable genuine reflection. Such reflection tends to cause conflict to emerge that patients have to work through if they are to take responsibility for those principles and values. Such reflection also leads to a development of life meaning in general. All this is where the values history comes in for the advance directive.

3 Negotiation of responsibility is a key way in which ethical meaning is worked through. As Jennifer Finch and Jennifer Mason note, in their work on responsibility in families, this begins to establish a moral identity even when there is no reference to values and principles (Finch and Mason, 1993). It is also a critical way of enabling collaboration between all the parties involved. Hence, it is key to the balancing of autonomies.

4 Autonomy emerges through this process as a more complex concept than has been suggested, summing up some of the aspects explored above:
   – Autonomy is not simply the result of someone taking a decision, not simply about freedom of choice. Autonomy is actually about authenticity, the person taking responsibility for their choices and values.
   – Autonomy involves the development of capacity and virtue. The person develops the capacity to think and feel through decisions.
   – Most importantly autonomy is not individualistic. As Al McFadyen puts it, a person only exists in relation to another, and communicates through dialogue. Identity and autonomy only emerge through that dialogue (McFadyen 1990). It is precisely

such dialogue which enables individuals not simply to clarify values and gain data but to find their own voice through the development of narrative as it emerges in relation to the different narratives in their life.

All this moves into a view of positive freedom, in addition to the negative freedom which seeks to protect the person from any manipulation or paternalism. Hence, rather than speaking of the term autonomy, it is possible to speak of 'shared governance', a governance of the self which accepts interdependence and mutual responsibility, leading to broader possible options.

In looking at the decision making process, Ardagh (1999) then suggests that doctors have to develop and apply 'moral imagination', literally putting themselves into the position of the patient. The final test for resuscitation, for instance, would be that in the light of identifying with the patient the doctor will answer the question 'Would I want this treatment?' In effect Ardagh is referring to empathy, the capacity to transcend the self and identify with the other (Robinson 2001, Chapter 2). This leads to a much more profound view of respect.

Respect is not based simply on respect for choice but rather on an awareness of the other and their life meaning and purpose. Such empathy is required not simply on the part of the doctor but on the part of the patient and family in the overall decision making process. The patient needs an empathy with the self to discern whether decisions are actually about denial, as Ryan (1996) would suggest. The family members need empathy if they are to understand the patient's value and life meaning.

Alongside the development of empathy is the development of trust in the medical practitioner – not simply as a competent doctor, but as someone who has heard and understood the values and purpose of the person and thus can attend to the non-medical factors which are part of any decisions.

The elements of decision making in clinical ethics are summed up in the following table devised by Jonsen and colleagues.

Box 4.1 *Elements of decision making in clinical ethics*

Medical indications

1 What is the patient's medical problem/history/diagnosis?

2 Is the problem acute/chronic/critical/emergent/reversible?

3 What are the goals of treatment?

4 What are the chances of success?

5 What are the plans in case of therapeutic failure?

6 In sum, how can this patient benefit from medical and nursing care, and how can harm be avoided?

Patient preferences

1 What has the patient expressed about preferences for treatment?

2 Has the patient been informed of benefits and risks, and understood and given consent?

3 Is the patient mentally capable and legally competent?

4 Has the patient expressed any prior preferences?

5 If incapacitated, who is the appropriate surrogate?

6 Is the patient unwilling or unable to co-operate with medical treatment?

7 In sum, is the patient's right to choose being respected to the extent possible in ethics and law?

Quality of life

1 What are the prospects, with or without treatment, for a return to the patient's normal life?

2 Are there biases that might prejudice the provider's evaluation of the patient's quality of life?

Contextual features

1 Are there family issues that might influence treatment decisions?

2 Are there provider issues (e.g. physicians and nurses) that might influence treatment decisions?

3 What physical, mental and social deficit is the patient likely to experience if treatment succeeds?

3 Are there financial and economic factors?

4 Is the patient's present or future condition such that continued life might be judged undesirable by them?

4 Are there religious or cultural factors?

5 Is there any plan or rationale to forgo treatment?

5 Is there any justification for breaching confidentiality?

6 What plans are there for comfort and palliative care?

6 Are there problems of allocation of resources?

7 What are the legal implications of treatment decisions?

8 Is clinical research or teaching involved?

9 Is there any provider or institutional conflict of interest?

Source: Jonson, A., Seigler, M., Winslade, W. (1998) *Clinical Ethics: A Practical Approach to Ethical Decisions in Clinical Medicine*, 4e. McGraw Hill, New York: 13.

The real world?

The decision making approach outlined above develops an autonomy which is much richer and satisfying than the simple consumer view. However, there are major questions. Firstly, if such a decision making process is used what would be the need for advance directives? Research would seem to indicate that advance directives do not make that much difference in practice. One study has found that advance directives make no real difference to the care in terms of patient satisfaction, personal wellbeing, survival time or quantity of drugs given (Sommerville

1996). The reasons for this are not clear, and could include a concern for equitable treatment, ignoring of advance directives, determination that an advance directive did not apply. Perhaps more importantly, this study indicates that where the patient was faced with the possibility of mental incapacity, through diseases such as AIDS, the dialogue which occurred before that incapacity was so intensive and profound that there was no need for dependence on advance directives (Sommerville 1996). If the process is right, then there will be no need for advance directives. This is much the argument for the care of the terminally ill. Through careful planning of care, and sharing of the values of hospice care in particular, patients can be enabled to retain dignity and autonomy throughout the experience, based on a relationship of trust. This may involve close relational work up to a time quite close to death.

The second question though, is how many people can expect this kind of treatment? This ideal of care is simply not there across the board.

- For some the critical problems arise suddenly and without a long term relationship with the medical staff.
- In the case of resuscitation there simply is not the time to gain the necessary data that enables professionals to hear the person's voice. The possibility of carrying cards is there but this too raise problems for the doctor in terms of judging whether it applies in the situation. Faced by this the concern for the safety of the patient overrides.
- Research suggests that practice in hospitals is not consistent in respect of dying patients. Mills and colleagues (1994) note that over half the patients in their research were competent and conscious until shortly before death but were unable to obtain minimal care interventions on a regular basis. The researchers concluded nursing contact was minimal and that there was 'distancing and isolation of patients' by all medical staff.

It is difficult to draw too many conclusions from research such as this. However, it highlights the fact this whole area of working through life meaning, values and treatment preferences with patients and families prior to death is very demanding and threatening for medical professionals. As we shall see in the next chapter, it raises major questions about treatment procedure, training and about team work with different professions.

In this real world it is clear that no approach can ensure exactly that the values, beliefs and wishes of the patient will be discovered and taken into account in every situation. Hence, the legal practice tends to stress broad approaches to decision making. A frequently used example of this is the 'Bolam' test, based on the case *Bolam v. Friern Hospital Management Committee* (1957) 2 A11 E.R. 118. This aims to reach a decision such as a 'reasonable' body of medical opinion would have made. This has been criticised precisely on the grounds that the decision may involve more than simple medical judgement (Musthill in *Re Bland* – see Case Study 3.3 on page 53). The case in *Re Conroy* (A2d 303 [NJ 1983]) applies more systems to decision making. The first of three stages looks for evidence of the patient's wishes. Failing such evidence the second stage looks to the balance of burdens and benefits. A third stage discontinues treatment if it is judged to be inhumane.

It must be stressed, however, that no system, test or standard can take away the need for the staff and family involved to develop moral discernment and empathy which will enable interpretation responsive to the needs of the particular situation.

Conclusions

In the light of all this debate we return to the case of John and that initial question as to how the advance directive would have affected the decision making process. In this case John did have an advance directive and the effect of it was important. At one level it added little to the actual data which the group had. In general terms it stated that he did not want intrusive and unnecessary treatment if he were in a state without mental capacity.

Where it was important was in the focusing of his voice. Empathy from the staff and family enabled John, literally, to participate in the conversation. The younger son was able to reflect on the values of his father and to begin to face up to and rethink the relationship he had with him before his father's dementia. Part of the reason why he was holding on to the 'new identity' of his father was precisely to avoid memories of his 'other father' and so to avoid the feelings of shame which he had developed. The directive enabled him to return to that father and begin to work through his relationship with him, and let go.

The oldest son was able to be reassured that he was not simply trying to 'get rid' of his father. Both had their perspectives reinforced by the evidence of the nursing staff who could point to the ambiguity of their father's condition. At times he did show great calmness, at other times he was clearly distressed. John's wife was able to let go and speak about him for the first time since the dementia had really taken hold. She shared how the whole experience had been like a death to her. She had lost her husband but was unable to grieve, having to put so much effort into support. She felt that now not even her support could sustain him.

The doctor had had little involvement in the case and for the most part looked to others, including the nurses, to guide her. However, while she knew that there was no hope of real recovery for John, she also felt that the decision was more than simply a medical one about withdrawing treatment. It was a matter of letting go and allowing the different members of John's life network to find their way of resolving their relationships with him.

This case begins to sum up many of the ethical questions that have emerged:

1 Autonomy cannot be seen simply as freedom of choice. The wishes of any one, at any time, have to be considered in the light of a given situation and of the relational network and their needs. Decision making for those patients who are not competent to make decisions themselves has to involve all those concerned.

2 This moves us away from a simple 'rights' view of ethics and more into 'virtue' or 'discourse' ethics. Virtue ethics stresses the importance of the community response. It is narrative based, and thus stresses the importance of the group working through their stories, and focuses in particular on the virtue of prudence or wisdom (McIntyre 1981). Wisdom is not simply about pragmatism but rather a genuine openness to the past, present and future (May 1994), and thus an openness to a common way through deciding about treatment. It also points to an ethic which is more about discourse (Habermas 1990, Nessa and Malterud 1999), enabling the development of dialogue that clarifies ethical and spiritual meaning, the development of trust, the recognition of shared values and the acceptance of different perspectives.

3 The concept of futile treatment cannot be used as the battleground for freedom versus paternalism. The attempt to find an objective medical definition is not possible, given the broader ethical concerns.

4 Attempts to use identity as the basis of a rights approach are inadequate, not least because identity itself is a social concept.

5 Respect for life remains important but is too general a concept to give specific guidance for this matter. The attempt to equate withdrawal of treatment with killing has no substance.

6 Ethical decision making is essentially social. This approach promotes shared governance and enables all parties to feel part of the decision and to begin to work through a moment of great transition in their lives. The focus then is not so much upon rights as upon right relationships, something close to the Jewish concept of Shalom. Shalom refers not simply to peace but also to right relationships, where the obligation to others in the significant community and beyond are addressed and responded to (Wilkinson 1998:21 and following).

Such a model, of course, is rarely totally put into practice. The constraints of time and relationships often mean that resolution of issues or relationships cannot be achieved. In which case decision making has to be based on best interest. Nonetheless, it is a model that can be aimed for and which requires team-work at all levels. The advance directive cannot of itself effect such resolution, but it can give the patient a voice in the process of deciding about treatment. At the very least then it can be encouraged by the medical and health care professions and can in itself, along with values histories, provide the basis for reflection on the patient's values and life meaning.

References

Ardagh, M. (1999) 'Resurrecting autonomy during resuscitation – the concept of professional substituted judgement.' *Journal of Medical Ethics*, 25: 375–378.

Armstong, J., Dixon, R., Robinson, S. (1999) *The Decision Makers: ethics for engineers*. Thomas Telford, London.

Asch, D., Hansen Fletcher, J., Lanken, P. (1995) 'Decisions to limit or continue life sustaining treatment by critical care physicians in the Unites States: conflicts between physicians' practices and patients' wishes.' *American Journal of Respiratory and Critical Care Medicine*, 151: 288–292.

Badham, P. (1998) 'Should Christians accept the validity of voluntary euthanasia?' In Gill, R. (ed.) *Euthanasia and the Churches*. Cassell, London.

Bauman, Z. (1993) *Postmodern Ethics*. Blackwells, Oxford.

Beauchamp, T., Childress, J. (2001) *Principles of Biomedical Ethics*, 5e. Oxford University Press, Oxford.

Berghams, R. (1998) 'Advance directives for non-therapeutic dementia research: some ethical and policy considerations.' *Journal of Medical Ethics*, 24: 32–37.

Berlin, I. (1969) 'Two concepts of liberty.' In Quinton, A. (ed.) *Political Philosophy*. Oxford University Press, Oxford.

Blackhall, L. (1987) 'Must we always use CPR?' *New England Journal of Medicine*, 315: 1347–1351.

Brett, A., McCullough L. (1986) 'When patients request specific interventions: defining the limits of the physician's obligations.' *New England Journal of Medicine*, 317: 1347–1351.

BMJ (2002) Editorial. *British Medical Journal*, 324: 629.

British Medical Association (1995) *Advance Statements about Medical Treatment, BMA Code of Practice*. BMJ, London.

Campbell, A. (1984) *Moderated Love*. SPCK, London.

Childress, J., Fletcher, J. (1994) 'Respect for autonomy.' *Hastings Center Report*, 24: 34–35.

Dworkin, R. (1993) *Life's Dominion: an argument about abortion, euthanasia and individual freedom*. Alfred Knopf, New York.

Finch, J., Mason, J. (1993) *Renegotiating Family Responsibilities*. Routledge, London.

Glick, S. (2000) 'The morality of coercion.' *Journal of Medical Ethics*, 26(5): 393–395.

Greaves, D. (1989) 'The future prospects for living wills.' *Journal of Medical Ethics*, 15: 179–182.

Halliday, R. (1997) 'Medical futility and the social context.' *Journal of Medical Ethics*, 23: 148–153.

Habermas, J. (1990) *Moral Consciousness and Communicative Action*. Polity Press, London.

Harris, J. (1985) *The Value of Life*. Routledge, London.

Healthcare Opposed to Euthanasia (1998) *Submission to the Lord Chancellor's Department*. HOPE, London.

Hope, T. (1996) 'Advance directives.' *Journal of Medical Ethics*, 22: 67–68.

Ikonomidis, S., Singer, P. (1999) 'Autonomy, liberalism and advance care planning.' *Journal of Medical Ethics*, 25: 522–527.

Jeffrey, P. (2001) *Going Against the Stream: ethical aspects of ageing and care*. Gracewing, Leominster.

John Paul II (1995) *Evangelium Vitae*. Vatican, Rome.

Jonson, A., Seigler, M., Winslade, W. (1998) *Clinical Ethics: a practical approach to ethical decisions in clinical medicine*. McGraw-Hill, New York.

Kennedy, I. (1997) 'Commentary 3: a response to Lowe.' *Journal of Medical Ethics*, 23: 161–163.

Kennedy, I., Grubb, A. (1994) *Medical Law: text with materials*, 2e. Butterworth, London.

Koehn, D. (1998) *Rethinking Feminist Ethics*. Routledge, London.

Kutner, L. (1969) 'Living wills.' *Indiana Law Journal*, 44: 539–554.

Loewy, E., Carlson, R. (1993) 'Futility and its wider implications.' *Archives of Internal Medicine*, 153: 429–431.

Luttrell, S., Sommerville, A. (1996) 'Limiting risks by curtailing rights: a response to Dr Ryan.' *Journal of Medical Ethics*, 22: 100–104.

Marriner-Tomey, A. (1993) *Transformational Leadership in Nursing.* Mosby-Year Book, St Louis.

Martin, D., Thiel, E., Singer, P. (1999) 'A new model of advance care planning.' *Archives of Internal Medicine,* 24: 19–21.

May, W. (1994) 'The virtues in a professional setting.' In Soskice, J. (ed) *Medicine and Moral Reasoning.* Cambridge University Press, Cambridge.

McFadyen, A. (1990) *Call to Personhood.* Cambridge University Press, Cambridge.

McIntyre, A. (1981) *After Virtue.* Duckworth, London.

Mills, M., Davies, H., Mcrae, W. (1994) 'Care of dying patients in hospital.' *British Medical Journal,* 309: 583–586.

Morgan, P., Lawton, P. (1996) *Ethical Issues in Six Religious Traditions.* Edinburgh University Press, Edinburgh.

Nedelsky, J. (1989) 'Reconceiving autonomy: sources, thoughts and possibilities.' *Yale Journal of Law and Feminism,* 1: 7–36.

Nelson, J. (1994) 'Families and futility.' *Journal of the American Geriatrics Society,* 42 (8): 879–882.

Nessa, J., Malterud, K. (1999) 'Tell me what's wrong with me: a discourse analysis approach to the concept of patient autonomy.' *Journal of Medical Ethics,* 24: 394–400.

Olick, R.S. (2001) *Taking Advance Directives Seriously: prospective autonomy and decisions near the end of life.* Georgetown University Press, Washington DC.

Parfit, D. (1979) 'Personal identity.' In Honderich, T., Burnyeat., M. (eds.) *Philosophy As It Is.* Pelican, Harmondsworth.

Pallis, C., Harley, D. (1995) *ABC of Brain Stem Death.* BMJ Publications, London.

Paris, J., Reardon, F. (1992) 'Physician refusal of requests for futile or ineffective interventions.' *Cambridge Quarterly for Healthcare Ethics,* 2: 127–134.

Robinson, S. (2001) *Agape, Moral Meaning and Pastoral Counselling.* Areus, Cardiff.

Rosner, F. (1994) 'Living wills.' *Lancet,* 343 (23 April): 1041.

Ryan, C. (1996) 'Betting your life: an argument against certain advance directives.' *Journal of Medical Ethics,* 22: 95–99.

Sandel, M. (1984) *Liberalism and its Critics.* New York University Press, New York.

Schneiderman, L., Jecker, N. (1993) 'Futility in practice.' *Archives of Internal Medicine,* 21(4): 437–441.

Schneiderman, L., Faber-Langendoen, F., Jecker, N. (1994) 'Beyond futility to an ethic of care.' *The American Journal of Medicine,* 96: 110–114.

Singer, P., Martin, D., Lavery, I., Thiel, E., Kelner, M., Mendelssohn, D. (1998) 'Reconceptualizing advance care planning from the patient's perspective.' *Archives of Internal Medicine,* 158: 879–884.

Society for the Protection of the Unborn Child (1998) *Beyond Autonomy: Response to the Green Paper 'Who Decides?'* SPUC, London.

Sommerville, A. (1996) 'Are advance directives really the answer? And what is the question? In Mclean, S. (ed.) *Death, Dying and the Law.* Dartmouth Publishing, Aldershot.

Warnock, M. (2002) 'Why patients need the right to die.' *The Guardian,* 30 April: 21.

Wilkinson, J. (1998) *The Bible and Healing.* Handsel Press, Edinburgh.

Wilson, L. (1999) *Living Wills.* Nursing Times Clinical Monograph, London.

Yong, G. (1995) *Respect for Human Life.* (Diocese of Singapore Pastoral Letter), Singapore.

Youngner, S. (1988) 'Who defines futility?' *Journal of the American Medical Association,* 260: 2094–2095.

5 From Theory to Practice

The purpose of this chapter is to bring together the themes we have discussed, and to explore how they impinge upon healthcare practice and delivery. This is particularly important because – whatever terms we use: 'living wills', 'advance directives' or 'advance statements' – all find their raison d'être at the cutting edge of care. For this reason, it is vital to place the defining features of these elements within the context and situation that characterise their application. In doing this, attention will be focused upon the following:

- Advance directives, decision making, and the legal context for the healthcare professional
- The defining features of a 'values history'
- The pragmatic considerations involved in making an advance directive.

Legal considerations: a summary

The proxy

Proposed legislation is focusing more on the role of the proxy in any decision making involving treatment for the patient who does not have the capacity to be involved in that decision. It is not clear when such legislation will be enacted, but will focus on the following issues:

- Enduring power of attorney will be extended. This will include the power to give authority for withdrawal of artificial nutrition and hydration only if so stated in the terms of the power of attorney.
- Managers (see page 50), if appointed by the Court of Protection, will not have that power; such prerogative will remain the gift of the Court.
- Evidence of competence at the time of making the power of attorney will be required.
- The continuing power of attorney (CPA) will have to be registered.
- Where the view of the attorney (CPA) differs from the medical practitioner, the court will be consulted.

At present, the ordinary power of attorney lasts for only as long as the person who gives the power has mental competence. Enduring power of attorney only applies to property. Nonetheless, it is accepted that the family should be consulted on decisions about refusal of treatment where the patient is incompetent. This has raised issues for single sex partnerships who have not been recognised as family. Hence, in 2000 the TUC Lesbian and Gay Conference asked the TUC to promote advance directives as a means of giving such partners more of a say. This was later enshrined in the TUC briefing of November 2001 which encourages those who make advance directives to nominate a 'health care proxy'. Whilst such proxies have no status in law, such a formal nomination would encourage medical practitioners to include them in the interpretation of the directive (TUC 2001).

Advance directives and decision making

In England and Scotland the conclusion is that common law should apply along with the use of codes of practice, such as the BMA Code (see Appendix I). While common law does not legislate directly for advance directives, it does confirm the principle of consent for treatment and therefore the importance of taking into account any advance directive from the patient. In Scotland, the Act specifically starts from the premise that the medical practitioner responsible for the incapacitated adult shall 'have authority to do what is reasonable in the circumstances, in relation to the medical treatment, to safeguard or promote the physical health of the adult' (Adults With Incapacity Act 2000, 47, 20).

A valid advance directive requires:

- Evidence that the person was competent at the time of writing it
- Evidence that the person is fully informed about the nature of their directive and its implications
- Evidence that the person has made the decision outlined in the advance directive without pressure or coercion
- Evidence that the directive has not been changed.

In making the decision, other factors need to be addressed by the medical practitioners. For example:

1 The advance directive should be examined in the light of the medical situation. In particular, if the directive is specific the doctor should determine whether it actually applies to that situation.

2 It should be determined whether or not the person is capable of making their own decisions. The test of capacity is summed up in the BMA Code. Age Concern note the importance of being sensitive to cultural differences in assessing capacity (Age Concern England 2002).

3 Circumstances that may have changed from the time of the initial directive should be explored. This includes new treatments.

4 Decision making should, when possible, be carried out in full consultation with the other medical staff and with the family of the patient.

5 The treatment of such patients should be carried out from the principle of best interest, something that routinely includes considering the patient's wishes.

6 No advance directive can require the doctor to do anything that is unlawful, including assisting suicide or practising euthanasia.

7 An advance directive will be superseded should it be in conflict with mental health legislation that seeks to protect the patient or others.

8 Where an advance directive is valid, applies to the situation and there are no indications that are contrary to it, it should be respected.

9 There will be no liability for health care workers in the law of tort if the patient's wishes about not following or withdrawing treatment are followed, and he or she dies, or if life-saving treatment precludes a long search for evidence of an advance directive.

10 Where there is doubt, life should be preserved in the case of an emergency. In the case of doubt where there is no emergency, legal opinion should be sought – in the first place through the Official Solicitor's office, and then through the courts.

11 Any dispute occurring between medical practitioners, or between medical practitioners and family, should also be referred to the courts. The Scottish Act makes provision for a nominated medical practitioner to give a second opinion. Where there is still dispute there may be an appeal to the Court of Session.

12 A medical practitioner who objects to any directive on grounds of conscience should declare this at once and offer the patient the

option of seeing another doctor. In the event of an emergency where no other doctor is available, the doctor then has a legal duty to comply with any appropriate advanced directive (refusal).

13 Where an advance directive, such as refusal of tube feeding, is accepted then care of the patient should be appropriate, ensuring warmth and shelter, management of distressing symptoms, and hygiene control.

14 There is no guidance from the law in the case of treatment during pregnancy. Each case would have to be examined separately and, where there is doubt about the applicability of an advance directive, legal advice should be sought.

15 If the doctor has reasonable ground for believing that there is an advance directive, where time permits this should be obtained. Emergency treatment should not be withheld while searching for an advance directive.

16 It will be the patient's responsibility for ensuring the advance directive is communicated to the doctor. This should be stored in the patient's medical records, and with any guardian or attorney. When the directive is given orally it should be noted in the records.

17 It may be that an advance directive is found after life prolonging treatment has been initiated. The BMA view is that this should not be grounds for not implementing the directive. 'Treatment should be discontinued in accordance with the directive once this is known', and once the directive has been validated, and confirmed by a proxy decision maker (BMA, guidance on advance statements, www.bma.org.uk/ap.nsf/Content/__Hub+ethics+publications).

In all this it is important to have in place a framework to ensure that every relevant view is taken account of. It would seem sensible that each health care trust should develop its own framework and protocol, in relation to BMA and GMC guidelines.

Jehovah's Witnesses

As noted above, a doctor is obliged to comply with a Jehovah's Witness's refusal of a blood transfusion where this refusal represents the patient's continuing wishes. The Witness does not intend to die, indeed has a conscientious objection to suicide, though may be aware of the possibility of death as the consequence of the refusal of treatment.

In this case the patient accepts this as a consequence, obeying their conscience, and this overrides any best interest arguments. Nonetheless, the doctor would need to be certain of the patient's wishes in practice, as well as of the grounds for those wishes, and thus be convinced that the patient had not been manipulated in any way. Raanan Gillon develops this in an important discussion in the *Journal of Medical Ethics* (Gillon 2000). Whilst any religious belief should be respected this does not preclude a challenge to justify such a belief rationally. He argues that in terms of a competent patient this might include giving the patient references for Jehovah's Witness writers who argue that there are no grounds for refusing blood transfusion. This may well be part of any decision making in drawing up an advance directive, or even be part of the decision making of the family or friends, especially where the views of the incompetent patient are not clear. This does not coerce patient or family. Rather, it simply adds to the reflective process.

Framing a values history

While the values history lacks any legal support or clarification, it is a useful means of clarifying the situation for doctors and families where there is time to reflect on the decision.

The values history might be worked through discursively in terms of vignettes. These simply give examples of clinical scenarios, about which the patient can share views and feelings. The use of vignettes is really a learning or communicative tool. It helps the patient to focus on treatment, on hopes and values, and should thus lead to greater clarity.

A good example of this is the Values History Statement devised by Chris Docker, based on work in Helsinki and Seattle, which acts as Section B of his Advance Medical Directive. In this, several different scenarios are set out detailing the chance for patients to indicate how they would feel about having to endure them. These include:

- Permanent paralysis, where the patient cannot interact with other people
- Permanent inability to 'speak meaningfully', though one can care for one's own daily needs

- Permanent inability to take care of oneself, being totally reliant on others in all things
- Permanent pain, which cannot be totally controlled by medication
- Experience of a short-term coma.

(Docker 1996)

Vignettes could also be created around severe dementia, persistent vegetative state (PVS) and so on.

Individuals are then asked to grade these according to how they feel about them (worse or not worse than death) and whether they would want life sustaining treatment. This is not meant to give specific guidance, but rather to demonstrate feelings and values.

A more detailed values history might be worked through in terms of an *extended values history form*. It is not necessary to use a form though it does have the advantage of helping patients to focus on the issues in question. Certain points are critical in the development of such a history:

1 It should emerge out of the dialogue with the doctor.
2 The work on values history should begin before a crisis occurs. It is easier to begin to focus on issues then not least because of a greater sense of control. It also provides the starting point of reflectivity. It might be advisable to present all patients at some point with such a form. How much they fill in is then up to them.
3 Consultation should be far and wide – family, friends, spiritual advisers etc.
4 The dialogue may take the person into much more profound reflection, not least because it will focus on illness, possible death and life meaning.

Docker offers one version of this form that asks basic questions under the following headings:

1 **Overall attitude towards life and health.** This can include life meaning and purpose, and the person's view of well being.
2 **Personal relationships.** This helps the patient to reflect on the most important relationships, and what part significant persons may play in his or her future medical treatment choices.
3 **Thoughts about independence and self-sufficiency.** This is a critical section that enables the doctor to see how the person feels about long-term dependency.

4 **Living environment.** What is the living environment that the person is most comfortable with?

5 **Religious background and beliefs.** Questions about these can help a person to focus on areas of belief that they have never really associated with health or illness. This need not be confined to organised religion.

6 **Thoughts about illness, dying and death.** These might range from what meaning might be found in dying and death to where the person would like to die.

7 **Finances.** Questions here look at the fears that may surround the cost of care.

8 **Funeral plans.** This encourages positive use of individuals' imagination to see how they might want their life to be remembered. This can extend even to thoughts about obituaries.

(Docker 1995)

What is most striking about such a form is its exhaustive nature. Such is its breadth that it is comparable to the work in psychology and spirituality looking into the part these areas play in informing health and health care (Miller 1999). These disciplines have looked at the different ways in which the spirituality of the patient might be assessed – trying to highlight and fulfil spiritual needs. The term 'spirituality' refers to the development of significant life meaning, inclusive of a person's cognitive and affective orientation towards a relational network. This can range from the self to others, the environment and God. While this can include religious faith it is not exclusively identified with it.

We would urge the different approaches and perspectives to come together, for two reasons. Firstly, if there are different forms assessing different areas it could become confusing for the patient. Secondly, the areas of overlap are immense. The sections on beliefs, values, relationships, death and dying are very much a focus of spirituality (Gorsuch and Miller 1999).

We would also urge the development of forms that are flexible, allowing individuals simply to begin by developing feelings and values in relation to their particular situation. This could include use in well man and well woman clinics, where there is a positive view of health. Such an approach would allow questions of death and dying to emerge later, and all as either part of the relationship with the doctor or arising from the actual context of the care. For many it is important not to consider the question of death until it becomes necessary. Much of this is about allowing patients to develop their own narrative, at their own pace and in response to their particular situation.

The idea of narrative is a hard one to keep within limits and a possible way through this is to develop some form of contract. This is analogous to the learning contract in education, or the counselling contract, where all involved are encouraged in verbal or written form to set down their basic expectations. Applied to medical care this enables the development of mutuality, allowing the patient to have input. It also clarifies the limitations, of patients, medical staff and of treatments. The contract also establishes trust and the possibility of developing dialogue. It is possible to revisit and modify such verbal contracts, all the while identifying and affirming not just rights but values (Robinson 2001).

Attempts to develop a contractual approach in the Patient's Charter were on the whole not successful. Part of the reason for this was the stress on rights rather than relationships. Because the contract is based in the medical relationship, and in response to the particular situation, it provides a neat framework in which to develop both the values history and the advance directive. Because it is relationship-based rather than legally binding it enables the development of trust. Only in the context of such a relationship can a patient begin to explore the major themes that surround living wills and values histories.

The themes of narrative and mutuality led the American Association of Retired Persons to pass over the use of a form in favour of simply writing down the fruits of dialogue about such questions as:

- 'How do you feel about your current health?'
- 'How important is independence and self-sufficiency in your life?'
- 'What role do religious beliefs play in you life?'
- 'What are your thoughts about life in general in its final stages: your hope and fears, enjoyments and sorrows?'
- 'How do you imagine handling illness, disability, dying and death, especially near the end of life?'
- 'How might personal relationships affect medical decision making, especially near the end of life?' (AARP 1995)

Another way of approaching this is to invite patients to reflect on their personal history and, in particular, on the network of relationships which give meaning to their life. This can range from the individual to community relationships, to the environment and the Divine. Through this reflection the basic values emerge and are clarified. This exercise tends to focus on faith (in relationships), purpose and self worth, as well as hope. In the light of these concepts, patients can be encouraged to reflect on the meaning that illness may have within their life.

There are several ways then of enabling value clarification and awareness, and the medical practitioner or pastoral care worker should not be constrained by any particular form but be able to use whatever way is most productive for the individual patient concerned.

Advance directives

Writing your own

Advance directives can be oral or written. Oral directives are quite sufficient, especially in a context where the patient and medical staff are in close contact, such as the hospice.

Written directives can be either on a pre-prepared form or in the person's own words. The BMA has offered a checklist for framing one's own words:

- Full name
- Address
- Name and address of general practitioner
- Whether advice was sought from health professionals
- Signature
- Date
- Witness signature
- A clear statement of your wishes, either general or specific
- If applicable the name, address and telephone number of the person you have nominated to be consulted about treatment decisions
- Date reviewed and signature. (BMA 1995:39)

In the light of the proposed legislation, this form of words does not of itself provide enough evidence of the living will having been worked through in an informed way. We would therefore recommend that, in addition, the general practitioner is asked to sign it to signify that full consultation between patient and doctor has occurred. Where the directive is an oral one, health professionals should be satisfied that the patient is fully informed.

The danger of writing one's own advance directive is that it is not effectively lodged, such that it can be referred to as quickly as possible. Hence, it is important to ensure that a copy is with the doctor and is recorded in the patient's notes, and that copies are with family and/or close friends. Once again it is important to have discussed the contents carefully with all who hold a copy of the directive.

Content and maintenance

The Patients' Association has usefully summed up key points that might be passed on to the patient about making and maintaining the advance directive:

- Remember that your advance directive can be general or specific or both
- Gather as much information as possible and discuss your views with relatives, health professionals and other people who are close to you
- Ensure that your wishes are clearly expressed and can be easily understood
- Check that you have complied with the formal requirements for your document
- Let people close to you know your decision: make sure your statement can be found when needed
- Plan to update or at least review your statement at regular intervals
- Consider naming someone to take part on your behalf in future decisions about your medical treatment (Patients' Association 1996:20).

Raising the issue

Raising the issue of advance directives with patients can, of course, be difficult. However, research shows patients, especially those over 65, do appreciate this. In one study the majority of those consulted said that they were interested in the concept, having had little previous knowledge of it; 92 per cent indicated that 'they would no longer wish their lives to be prolonged by medical interventions' (Schiff, Rajkmur, Bulpitt 2000:1640).

As with the values history, we would suggest that the issue of advance directives should be raised sensitively and in the context of the ongoing medical history and the therapeutic relationship. The doctor is in a difficult position, being a medical expert who can advise about options and consequences, but not always trained in the non-directive techniques that would ensure the patient's autonomy is developed and maintained. It is particularly important, therefore, that the doctor is able to communicate clearly and effectively about the nature of any illness and the possible consequences. Admission to hospital is an anxious time, and therefore on the whole not the best time to raise this issue. However, it may be appropriate to raise the question of advance directives at this point with patients who might require cardiopulmonary resuscitation, such as those at risk of cardiac or respiratory failure. Once again, this can emerge out of sensitive reflection on the person's condition.

Above all, health professionals should try to avoid any pressure and ensure that there is no pressure from others. In this respect, doctors and other health professionals can help the person to think through the pros and cons of the advance directive, not least to demonstrate a degree of impartiality.

There is in all this an important balance between the patient's rights and wishes, and the perhaps more fundamental concern of the patient about the possibility of death. The one requires careful reflection and possibly advocacy on the part of health care staff. The other requires careful pastoral provision, not least because of the issue of mortality which, rather than freedoms or rights, might be foremost in the patient's mind.

The healthcare team

It is important to stress that though the role of the doctor tends to dominate discussions about advance directives, not least because of questions about refusal of treatment, there are important roles for all who are working in healthcare or community support. This raises the importance of flexible and effective teamwork, between nurses, counsellors, religious advisors and all who work with the elderly.

Often the nurse will be in a position of privilege, being close to the patient, yet still essentially a stranger. Hence, Stiles (1997) can write of the nurse as the 'shining stranger', who is there for the patient and the family at this time. Campbell (1984:49) writes of the nurse as providing skilled companionship. The nurse is often privy to unformed values histories, simply through sharing the patient's story. Because of this the nurse can be aware of the fears and hopes of the patient in a way not always possible for the doctor. This allows the nurse to begin conversations about present and future treatment, and about the patient's wishes for this. In the light of this the nurse can enable the patient to begin effective articulation of and planning for advance directives. The Royal College of Nursing recognises this and was involved in the development of the BMA (1995) Code of Practice.

Linda Wilson adds that evidence of an advance directive can also provide a very effective way for the nurse to begin talking about 'end of life issues' with the patient. In doing that she notes that nurses 'can achieve the following:

- Exploring with patients their concerns and worries and correcting any misconceptions
- Providing more opportunity for patient's to fully participate in their care planning
- Taking up the role of patient advocate and helping patients to avoid futile interventions not acceptable to them
- Developing trust and an understanding of the patient's wishes
- Enabling the patient to have a dignified death free of unnecessary intervention
- Helping return control to the patient' (Wilson 1999:9).

Wilson usefully reminds us that doctors and nurses should not act as witnesses to advance directives.

Religious leaders or spiritual advisers, especially hospital chaplains, may be able to provide space for the person to work through issues, and patients may well wish to clarify religious or quasi-religious feelings and ideas. Once again this helps the patient to work through important value clarification, and can act as the trigger to framing an advance directive. The same is true of counsellors, and any community or support organisation workers.

When patients begin to work through their values and feelings, issues to do with families and friends are inevitably raised. Healthcare professionals can help patients to involve family and friends in this reflection, not least through outlining their possible roles in relation to proxy decision making.

Figure 5.1 gives an example of an advance directive (statement) from within the UK; it was designed by the Patients' Association in conjunction with the British Medical Association. An American example of the Living Will and Health Care Proxy is offered in Appendix II.

Conclusions

Finding a voice for those who are mentally or physically incapacitated and so unable to give contemporaneous consent to treatment is, in essence, person-centred. Codes and laws are there to ensure that it remains so, rather than to be followed slavishly. Nothing can get away from the requirement of all those in the situation to make decisions and to do so with integrity, faithfulness and veracity; hence, the need as much for practical wisdom (*prudentia*) as for forms or codes.

At the centre of that, the advance directive allows the patient's voice to be part of the on-going dialogue (Emmanuel 2000). It is not a voice that must be obeyed without question. On the contrary the law sets up relationships and requirements which will test that voice just as the voice of the medical practitioner or attorney should be tested and worked through. Hence, this is not a simple matter of rights, or of autonomy versus paternalism. If there is a central right in this debate it is the right to be heard. This in turn enables real discussion between all who have an interest.

Such a right enables the dignity of the patient to be maintained, and the fears and hopes of the patient's family to be addressed. As Sommerville (1996:36) notes, that dignity can extend beyond personal wishes to authorising statements that are concerned for others, such as elective ventilation for organ donation.

At the heart of this is empathy, and moral and spiritual imagination. Any advanced directive will be judged on how it enables each of these to flourish.

Figure 5.1 Advance Statement (Patient's Association/BMA 1996) (page 1)

Advance statement about future medical treatment

(Complete as many sections as you wish. Delete any part of this document you want to exclude from your statement.)

TO MY FAMILY, MY MEDICAL PRACTITIONERS, OTHER HEALTH CARE PROFESSIONALS, AND ALL OTHER PERSONS CONCERNED.

I (Name) ....

of (Address) ....

....

....

make this Advance Statement of my wishes about future medical treatment in case I become unable to communicate these wishes by virtue of physical or mental incapacity. I am of sound mind and have arrived at the following decisions after careful consideration.

1 In respect of medical treatment in general:

a) **IF** – I have a serious physical illness from which there is no reasonable expectation of recovery, and in which my life is sustainable only by medical intervention treatment or artificial means, I do not wish to be subjected to medical intervention, the purpose of which is to solely prolong my life.

b) **IF** – I suffer from severe and permanent mental impairment, and my physical condition is such that medical treatment is required to keep me alive, I do not wish to receive that treatment.

c) **IF** – I become permanently unconscious with no likelihood of regaining consciousness, I do not wish to be kept alive by artificial means.

I nevertheless expect, in the circumstances described, any distressing symptoms (including any caused by the lack of fluid) to be actively controlled by appropriate palliative care, ordinary nursing care, analgesia or other treatments, even though some of these treatments may have the effect of shortening my life.

2 In respect of specific treatments:
(Please consult your doctor before completing this section)

I have been told that I have been diagnosed as suffering from:

....

....

I have the following wishes about medical treatment or investigations:

....

....

3 I have asked the following person to take part in decisions about my medical care on my behalf, if I am unable to speak for myself.

I have discussed my views about future medical treatment with him/her, and given him/her a copy of this document.

I wish him/her to be consulted about these decisions, and I ask those caring for me to respect the views he/she expresses on my behalf:

Name ....

Address ....

....

....

Telephone number ....

I, the undersigned, agree to act as the nominated representative of

....

Signature ....

Date ....

4 I have given copies of this statement to:

a) Name ....

Address ....

....

....

Figure 5.1 Advance Statement (page 2)

b) Name ....

Address ....

....

....

c) Name ....

Address ....

....

....

5 Additional requests and/or information

....

....

....

THIS DOCUMENT REMAINS EFFECTIVE UNTIL I MAKE IT CLEAR THAT MY WISHES AND DIRECTIVES HAVE CHANGED.

Signature ....

Date ....

I testify that the above-named signed this statement in my presence and made it clear to me that he/she fully understands what it means.

I do not know of any pressure brought on him/her to make such a statement and I believe it was made by his/her own wish. So far as I am aware, I am not a beneficiary under the terms of his/her ordinary will.

Witnessed by ....

Signature ....

Full name ....

Address ....

....

....

Figure 5.1 Advance Statement (page 3)

References

Age Concern England (2002) *Policy Position Paper on Capacity and Consent*, Age Concern England Policy Unit, London.

American Association of Retired Persons (1995) *Shape Your Health Care Future with Health Care Advance Directives*. Available on www.ama-assn.org. Reproduced in this book as Appendix II.

British Medical Association (1995) *Advance Statements about Medical Treatment: Code of Practice with Explanatory Notes*. BMA, London.

Campbell, A. (1984) *Moderated Love*. SPCK, London.

Docker, C. (1995) *Extended Values History Form*. Available on www.euthanasia.org/vh.html.

Docker, C. (1996) *Living Will*. Voluntary Euthanasia Society Scotland, Edinburgh.

Emmanuel, L. (2000) 'How living wills can help doctors and patients talk about dying' *British Medical Journal* 320:1618–1619.

Gillon, R. 'Refusal of potentially life saving blood transfusions by Jehovah's Witnesses: should doctors explain that not all JWs think it's religiously required' *Journal of Medical Ethics* 26(5), 299–301.

Gorush, R., Miller, W. (1999) 'Assessing Spirituality.' In Miller, W. (ed) *Integrating Spirituality into Treatment*. American Psychological Association, Washington DC.

Miller, W. (1999) *Integrating Spirituality into Treatment*. American Psychological Association, Washington DC.

Patients' Association/British Medical Association (1996) *Advance Statements About Future Medical Treatment*. Patients' Association, London.

Robinson, S. (2001) *Agape, Moral Meaning and Pastoral Counselling*. Aureus, Cardiff.

Schiff, R., Rajkumar, C., Bulpitt, C. (2000) 'Views of elderly people on living wills: interview study' *British Medical Journal* 320: 1640–1641.

Sommerville, L. (1996) 'Are advance directives really the answer? And what was the question?' In McLean, S. (ed.) *Death, Dying and the Law*. Dartmouth Publishing, Aldershot.

Stiles, M. (1997) 'The shining stranger: nurse–family spiritual relationships.' *Cancer Nursing*, 13 (4): 235–245.

Wilson. L. (1999) *Living Wills*. Nursing Times Books, London.

TUC *Living Wills*. www.tuc.org.uk/equality/tuc-3973-f0.cfm.

Appendix I:
British Medical Association Code of Practice concerning Advance Statements and Medical Treatment

(Reproduced in full by kind permission)

Advance Statements about Medical Treatment – Code of Practice. Report of the British Medical Association, April 1995

Preface to Advance Statements About Medical Treatment

In 1997, the Government for England and Wales announced that it believed there to be a clear need for reform of the law to improve and clarify decision making processes for people unable to make decisions for themselves, or people who cannot communicate their decisions. It based this view on the extensive work the English Law Commission had undertaken in the preceding six years. The Law Commission had investigated and proposed improvements to the law in this area, including a proposal to introduce legislation to put advance directives on a statutory footing. This was one of the issues on which the Government consulted in 1997.

The BMA's code of practice on advance decision making came about in response to a call for guidance from the House of Lords Select Committee on Medical Ethics.[1] Published two years before the Government's consultation, it describes the common law and the BMA's views on advance decisions. It includes advice on drafting and implementation, and describes the responsibilities of health professionals. It has sold over 4000 copies, and in excess of 13,000 summaries have been distributed.

---

1 British Medical Association (1995) *Advance Statements about Medical Treatment*. London, BMA.

Following its consultation, the Government in October 1999 published detailed proposals for law reform.[2] The Lord Chancellor's Department stated its intention to legislate to give statutory recognition to the definitions of capacity and best interests, and to clarify the basis on which decisions may be made on behalf of incapacitated adults. It also proposed to make provision for the appointment of proxies entitled to take medical treatment decisions. Advance directives, however, are not part of the legislative plans. Instead, the Government published a clear statement of the present legal position.

'The current law and medical practice is as follows. It is a general principle of law and medical practice that all adults have the right to consent to or refuse medical treatment. Advance statements are a means for patients to exercise that right by anticipating a time when they may lose the capacity to make or communicate a decision.

'Adults with capacity have the right to refuse or withdraw their consent to medical treatment. We do not accept that the decision has either to be reasonable or has to be justified to anyone apart from the individual who is making the decision. It follows that the Government respects the right of people with capacity to be able to define, in advance, which medical procedures they will and will not consent to at a time when that individual has become incapable of making or communicating that decision.'

The Government went on to cite the legal cases in which the courts have approved this principle. It also reported that response to its consultation exercise showed a wide range of views on what is a complex and sensitive subject. Some people believe that advance statements are morally wrong and tantamount to euthanasia. Others see them as a natural extension of the rights of individuals to make decisions for themselves. Given the division of opinion and the flexibility inherent in developing case law, the Government chose not to legislate at the present time. It made the following statement.

---

2 Lord Chancellor's Department (October 1999) *'Making Decisions': The Government's Proposals for Making Decisions on Behalf of Mentally Incapacitated Adults*. London, HMSO.

'The Government is satisfied that the guidance contained in case law, together with the Code of Practice Advance Statements About Medical Treatment published by the British Medical Association, provides sufficient clarity and flexibility to enable the validity and applicability of advance statements to be decided on a case by case basis. However, the Government intends to continue to keep the subject under consideration in the light of future medical and legal developments.'

In Scotland, there has been a similar process which has led to the Adults with Incapacity (Scotland) Act 2000. Consultation papers to discuss the scope of legislation have made some reference to advance directives, but the Act makes no reference to these. In other words, a policy decision to omit advance directives has again been made.

The BMA believes that limited legislation to translate the common law into statute and clarify the non-liability of doctors who act in accordance with an advance statement would be helpful. In the absence of this, however, we welcome the Government's statement of the legal position and recognition of the BMA's Code of Practice.

Dr Michael Wilks
Chairman, BMA Medical Ethics Committee
4 April 2000

Part I – Background

1 Introduction

This guidance is a response to the House of Lords Select Committee on Medical Ethics, which in 1994 called for a Code of Practice on advance directives for health professionals. A multi-professional group under the aegis of the British Medical Association and medical and nursing Royal Colleges undertook the task of drafting it. Oral and written evidence was received from a wide range of individuals and groups. We wish to thank them for their help.

The Code takes a broad and essentially practical approach. It considers a range of advance statements, rather than limiting itself to those which have 'directive' force. It advises that there are both benefits and dangers to making treatment decisions in advance. Health professionals and patients should be aware of both. Nevertheless, carefully discussed advance statements have an important place in the development of a genuinely more balanced partnership between patients and health professionals. inevitably, the concept of shared decision making implies a renegotiation of the traditional scope of clinical discretion in favour of accommodating patients' views. This is part of a growing trend of people taking greater personal responsibility for their health. It is to be welcomed.

Special importance attaches to a person's desire to make the manner of their dying consistent with the pattern of their life.

But sensitive and compassionate management of death is only one aspect of a longer dialogue about choice which should occur between those giving and those needing health care. The Code does not restrict advance statements to discussions about death but recognises their potential value in other situations where people wish to influence what happens to them after the onset of mental incapacity. Nevertheless, advance statements appear to have only limited value in relation to the treatment of recurrent episodic mental illness. This is a unique area in which patients are unable to refuse the compulsory detention and treatment for mental disorder authorised by mental health legislation, although notice of their preferred treatment options may be helpful.

We endorse the recommendation of the Select Committee that health professionals should have training appropriate to their ethical responsibilities. Training must include the skills of sensitive communication and receptivity. Sensitive, continuing dialogue is given high priority, for example, in the palliative care setting which provides some effective models of oral advance statements.

1.1 This Code reflects good clinical practice in encouraging dialogue about individuals' wishes concerning their future treatment. It does not address euthanasia, assisted suicide or methods for allocating health service resources. These are entirely separate from advance statements.

1.2 At all stages of life, timely discussion of treatment options is an important part of the duty of care owed by health professionals to those who consult them. Recognising and respecting the individual patient's values and preferences are fundamental aspects of good practice.

The Code seeks to divorce 'advance directives' from practices of euthanasia and assisted suicide and places statements and directives within an accepted framework of discussion and communication.

2 Definitions

2.1 Advance statements: People who understand the implications of their choices can state in advance how they wish to be treated if they suffer loss of mental capacity. Just as adults must be consulted about treatment options, young people under the age of majority (age 18) are entitled to have their views taken into account. An advance statement (sometimes known as a living will) can be of various types (see also Figure 1):

- A requesting statement reflecting an individual's aspirations and preferences. This can help health professionals identify how the person would like to be treated without binding them to that course of action, if it conflicts with professional judgement.
- A statement of the general beliefs and aspects of life which an individual values. This provides a summary of individual responses to a list of questions about a person's past and present wishes and future desires. It makes no specific request or refusal but attempts to give a biographical portrait of the individual as an aid to deciding what he or she would want.
- A statement which names another person who should be consulted at the time a decision has to be made. The views expressed by that named person should reflect what the patient would want. This can supplement and clarify the intended scope of a written statement but the named person's views are presently not legally binding in England and Wales. In Scotland, the powers of a tutor dative may cover such eventualities.
- A clear instruction refusing some or all medical procedures (advance directive). Made by a competent adult, this does, in certain circumstances, have legal force.
- A statement which, rather than refusing any particular treatment, specifies a degree of irreversible deterioration (such as a diagnosis of

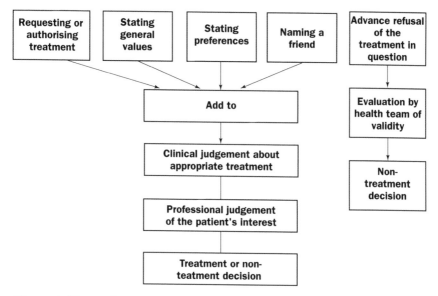

Figure 1: Types of advance statement (living will)

persistent vegetative state) after which no life sustaining treatment should be given. For adults, this again can have legal force.

- A combination of the above, including requests, refusals and the nomination of a representative. Those sections expressing clear refusal may have legal force in the case of adult patients.

An advance statement can be a written document, a witnessed oral statement, a signed printed card, a smart card or a note of a discussion recorded in the patient's file. Only a clear refusal of particular treatment by an adult has potential legal force. Clear general statements of preferences should be respected if appropriate but are not legally binding. Any advance statement (whether a consent or refusal, written or oral) is superseded by a clear and competent contemporaneous decision by the individual concerned. In the case of young people under the age of majority (age 18), advance statements should be taken into account and accommodated if possible but can be overruled by a court or a person with parental responsibility.

Medical treatment decisions are seldom choices made once for all time but involve a series of steps as a patient's clinical condition changes and his or her understanding of the real and potential implications develops. Profoundly life-affecting treatment decisions are often made against a background of uncertainty, since medicine itself is uncertain and because new techniques are constantly evolving.

The progress or remission of a disease can be affected by physiological or psychological factors unique to the individual. Each stage of treatment involves discussion between patients and health professionals. Loss of mental capacity robs people of the opportunity to participate in the dialogue or to re-assess their options. Advance statements are an imperfect substitute, but for some they are the only means of expressing their wishes about what they want to happen.

2.2 Advance directives (refusals): Competent, informed adults have an established legal right to refuse medical procedures in advance. An unambiguous and informed advance refusal is as valid as a contemporaneous decision. Health professionals are bound to comply when the refusal specifically addresses the situation which has arisen. Refusal is a serious matter, ideally to be considered in discussion with health professionals.

Since no-one can demand that medical treatment be given, statements purporting to 'direct' or instruct health professionals are necessarily refusals. Although a clear refusal is potentially legally binding, a refusal seriously likely to affect other people adversely (such as exposing them to the risk of harm) may be invalidated. This includes a refusal of basic care.

Competent adults have an established legal right to reject medical advice, assessment or treatment, except in cases where this harms others or conflicts with legislation (see Section 4).

What can be refused contemporaneously can also be refused in advance. All advance decisions carry some risk of error in evaluating possible future events and feelings. The legally binding nature of a competent advance refusal may increase the gravity of the risk. When people decide to take on these risks, it is important that health professionals provide factual information to help them (see Section 6). Young people under the age of majority cannot make legally binding treatment refusals although their wishes should be taken into consideration.

2.3 Care: Basic care means those procedures essential to keep an individual comfortable. The administration of medication or the performance of any procedure which is solely or primarily designed to proved comfort to the patient or alleviate that person's pain, symptoms or distress are facets of basic care. In each case, health professionals must continually assess the scope of measures essential for the patient's comfort. Although the law on this matter is not clear, this Code proves that as a matter of public policy, people should not be able to refuse basic care in advance or instruct others to refuse on their behalf (see also Section 5).

The adult patient's right to refuse medical interventions is well recognised by the common law. There are no clearly defined limits as to the sort of care or treatment which an informed, competent adult can refuse. Statutory powers under public health and mental health legislation, however, recognise a public interest in limiting in exceptional cases an individual's freedom to refuse medical examination and hospitalisation. These laws are based on the presumption that people cannot exercise their freedom in a manner which puts others at risk of harm. The Code reflects the view that a certain minimal level of intervention ('basic care') should be given notwithstanding a patient's refusal, since failure to do so exposes nurses, doctors and possibly other patients to unacceptable harms or burdens.

Defining 'basic care' is problematic. A definition too tightly drawn may lead to unintentional omissions, whereas a definition which is too wide gives rise to uncertainty. In the face of an apparently valid refusal of all interventions, the Code recommends that only those measures essential for patient comfort can be given. These will require constant reappraisal in each individual case and attention must be paid to the individual's verbal and non-verbal indications of his or her comfort needs. It is generally accepted that basic care includes warmth, shelter, pain relief, management of distressing symptoms, such as breathlessness and vomiting, and hygiene measures, such as management of incontinence. Recognising that near the end of life, patients seldom want nutrition or hydration, basic care would nevertheless include measures such as moistening a patient's mouth as necessary for comfort.

This is a controversial area where lawyers and courts may differ. The Code advises that since the comfort of the mentally incapacitated person is the prime criterion, appropriate food or drink should be made available for (but not forced upon) those who manifest a clear desire for it. The implication of this recommendation is that an advance refusal of oral feeding can be withdrawn by a person who retains sufficient mental capacity to indicate a desire for it. Nutrition and hydration should not be given to a person who indicates opposition. Invasive measures such as tube feeding should not be instituted contrary to a clear advance refusal.

In cases of disagreement or the need for greater clarity on the issue of refusal of basic care in an individual case, application should be made to the courts for clarification.

2.4 Capacity: Indicates an ability to understand the implications of the particular decision which the individual purports to make. The High Court has held that a person has capacity if he or she can understand and retain the information relevant to the decision in question, can believe that information and can weigh that information in the balance to arrive at a choice[1]. (For assessment of capacity, see Section 8).

'Capacity' is a legal term. Capacity and competence are used interchangeably in this document. People who lack the ability to understand the ramifications of financial decisions, for example, may well understand the implications of medical treatment. A distinction is drawn between an ability to understand and the fact of having actually understood. People who possess the ability may make an invalid decision if it has not been explained in a manner they can be said to have understood. Although they may understand and weigh the implications, young people under the age of majority do not have the same rights at law as an adult (see Section 4).

Part II – Making treatment choices

3 Making treatment choices

3.1 Adults can refuse clinical procedures contemporaneously or in advance of deteriorating mental capacity. Although no parallel right to insist upon a specific procedure or to order one of various treatment options is recognised in law, dialogue with patients about the choices facing them is an essential part of ethical health-care. Patients may properly expect to be provided with the details they need in an accessible form to allow them to make informed choices.

Statements expressing requests or preferences are not legally binding but should be respected and complied with if appropriate. Patients may prefer not to make a legalistic document but to talk to a doctor or nurse about their wishes and have these reflected in their notes. In such cases, patients should be encouraged to check the notes made about them to ensure they agree with what is written.

3.2 Discussion of options should be responsive to a patient's actual anxieties rather than trying to shape the patient's wishes to a preconceived standard format.

Patients may feel it is less threatening to talk about future options in a GP or outpatient setting. Continuous discussion, noted in the patient record, is a pattern which has developed in British palliative care services. Although we recognise there may be value in developing a standard format for advance statements, in practice this would be likely to undervalue those alternative methods for expressing preferences, including an oral statement.

3.3 Many personal, non-clinical issues influence how competent people reach decisions. When decisions are made on behalf of people who cannot choose for themselves, their previously expressed wishes and values should be taken into account. It is principally for the individual to decide what is right for him or herself. The best outcome from a clinical perspective, although an important part of the evaluation, is seldom the sole consideration for an individual. Health professionals have legal and ethical obligations to act in the best interests of those for whom they have undertaken a duty of care. Judgement of what constitutes an individual's best interests rests upon the ascertainable past and present wishes and feelings of the individual as well as clinical factors.

3.4 An advance directive is not restricted to care in hospital. It may also cover care at home, in a nursing home or in a hospice. There may be misapprehensions that advance directives (refusals), which can have legal force, only apply in certain locations or if counter-signed by a doctor as witness. No such requirements are recognised at common law.

4 The legal position

4.1 Common law establishes that an informed refusal of treatment made in advance by an adult who understands the implications of that decision has the same legal power as a contemporaneous refusal. In order to be legally binding, the individual must have envisaged the type of situation which has subsequently arisen. In all circumstances, a contemporaneous decision by a competent individual overrides previously expressed statements by that person.

4.1.1 Consent and treatment refusal: A conscious, mentally competent adult cannot be given treatment without his or her valid consent. Consent may not be valid if insufficient relevant information is given. It is illegal and unethical to treat an adult who is capable of understanding and willing to know, unless the nature of the procedure, its purpose and implications have been explained and that person's agreement obtained.

The right to refuse screening, diagnostic procedures or treatment can be for reasons which are 'rational, irrational or for no reason'.[2] The Court of Appeal held in 1992 that an adult is entitled to refuse treatment, irrespective of the wisdom of that decision.[3] For the refusal to be valid, however, health professionals must be satisfied that the patient's capacity at the time of deciding was not affected by illness, medication, false information or pressure from other people (see Section 8 for assessing mental capacity). Discussing the legal duties of health professionals in relation to a patient's refusal of treatment Lord Donaldson stated that:

> 'Doctors faced with a refusal of consent have to give very careful and detailed consideration to the patient's capacity to decide at the time when the decision was made. it may not be the simple case of the patient having no capacity because, for example, at that time he had hallucinations. It may be the more difficult case of reduced capacity at the time when his decision was made. What matters is that the doctors should consider whether at that

time he had capacity which was commensurate with the gravity of the decision which he purported to make. The more serious the decision, the greater the capacity required. If the patient had the requisite capacity, they are bound by his decision. If not, they are free to treat him in what they believe to be his best interests'.[4]

4.1.2 Advance consent: Some advance statements provide not only for refusal of treatment but for the option of asking 'to be kept alive for as long as reasonably possible using whatever forms of treatment are available'. To the extent that they demand the continuation of futile treatment or treatment which the health care team can no longer justify as serving the patient's best interests, they have no legal force. They may also permit personal requests such as preservation of life until a particular nominated person can be called to the bedside to say goodbye. One of the important points about this type of statement is that it shows that advance decision making concerns a right to choose rather than a right to die.

4.1.3 Advance refusal: Adults who are capable of making current medical decisions for themselves can, if properly informed of the implications and con sequences, also refuse in advance medical treatment which might be necessary when their capacity will be impaired. In the Bland case,[5] Lord Goff of Chieveley said 'it has been held that a patient of sound mind may, if properly informed, require that life support should be discontinued. The same principle applies where the patient's refusal to give his consent has been expressed at an earlier date, before he became unconscious or otherwise incapable of communicating it'.

The patient must have possessed insight into the implications of refusing treatment at the time of making the advance refusal in order for it to be valid. It is irrelevant whether the refusal is contrary to the views of most other people or whether the person lacks insight into other aspects of life as long as he or she is able to decide on the one matter in question. When a Broadmoor patient refused amputation of his gangrenous foot, the High Court held this to be a valid refusal currently and for the future, despite the fact that the man held demonstrably erroneous views on other matters.[6]

4.2 Young people under the age of majority do not have the same rights at law as adults. it is good practice, however, for children and young people to be kept as fully informed as possible about their care and treatment. The Children Act 1989 emphasises that the views of minors should be sought and taken into account in matters which touch on their welfare. Where appropriate, they should be encouraged to take decisions jointly with those with whom they have a close relationship, especially parents.

Competent patients of any age should feel confident that their views count and are respected. Children and young people do not have the same legal rights as adults and should be informed that, although efforts will be made to meet their wishes, in cases of disagreement about measures conducive to their welfare their own views will not necessarily be determinative. Discussion with young people should be structured so as to help them identify their own wants and needs but they should also be encouraged to take decisions jointly with those with whom they have a close relationship, especially parents.

4.3 Advance statements are not covered by legislation. In cases of conflict with other legal provisions, advance statements are superseded by existing statute. The terms of the mental Health Acts take precedence and must prevail regarding treatment for mental disorder. A compulsorily detained adult can make a legally binding advance refusal of treatment not covered by the mental health legislation. Where appropriate, patients' preferences should be included in treatment plans for both informal and detained patients.

There is no statute on advance statements although common law recognises the legal force of advance directives (refusals of treatment). Nevertheless even clear and specific advance directives (refusals) are superseded by existing Acts of Parliament. Conflict might arise between an advance directive, which would otherwise be legally binding, and the legal authority to give treatment under the Mental Health Acts. The provisions of the Mental Health Act 1983, Mental Health (Scotland) Act 1984, and the Mental Health (Northern Ireland) Order 1986 authorise the assessment of individuals, their admission to hospital or to guardianship and if necessary medical treatment or care without their consent. A patient may be compulsorily admitted to hospital under the Act where it is necessary:

- In the interests of his or her own health
- Or in the interests of his or her own safety
- Or for the protection of other people.[7]

Any provisions of advance directives refusing treatment of mental illness are rendered invalid in circumstances where the patient is legally detained for treatment.

Treatment under the Mental Health Act 1983 in England and Wales is covered by guidance given in the Code of Practice,[8] Chapter 15 of which discusses the principles of patient consent in the context of treatment for mental disorder. It emphasises the importance of treatment plans for both informal and detained patients, including advice about the desirability, wherever possible, of discussing the whole plan with the patient. Patients' advance statements or preferences regarding treatment options should also be included in the plan and in the discussion of immediate and long-term goals. Any part of an advance statement or directive (refusal) which refers to medical treatment outside the scope of the mental health legislation requires careful consideration.

5 Public policy

5.1 Advance statements refusing basic care and maintenance of an incompetent person's comfort should not, as a matter of public policy, be binding on care providers. Although the law on this matter is not free from doubt, this Code provides that people should not be able to refuse basic care in advance or instruct others to refuse it on their behalf.

Personal autonomy, although important, cannot always be an overriding ethical principle. In most situations, the individual's right to refuse treatment outweighs any competing interests, including the wishes of other people. In exceptional circumstances, the individual's choice has unacceptable consequences, such as potentially serious harm for others which is sufficient to outweigh the patient's right of refusal. Others may be harmed if refusal of basic care leads, for example, to the spread of infection.

Caring for a person whose pain or symptoms are not sufficiently relieved as a result of an advance refusal may impose an intolerable burden on those around them, and abandonment of an incapacitated person is unacceptable.

Our view, that individuals cannot validly refuse basic care, does not necessarily imply that health professionals are obliged to provide every facet of basic care. They should, rather, provide that which is reasonable in the circumstances. Some patients are prepared to tolerate a degree of discomfort and reduced medication, for example, in order to remain sufficiently alert to enjoy the company of visitors. Particularly in a palliative care setting, medical and nursing procedures are continually adjusted to suit the patient's requirements without infringing upon those of other patients or carers.

5.2 In the absence of an advance statement by a person who is now incapable of deciding, health professionals have a duty to act in that person's best interests.

5.3 Relatives' views may help in clarifying a patient's wishes but relatives' opinions cannot overrule those of the patient or supplant health professionals' duty to assess the patient's best interest.

The assessment of a person's best interests includes consideration of what he or she would have wanted, if that can be discerned from people close to the patient or from previous remarks recorded in the patient's notes (see also Section 10 on implementation).

Part III – Drafting

6 *Making an advance statement*

6.1 Although oral statements are equally valid if supported by appropriate evidence, there are advantages to recording one's general views and firm decisions in writing. Advance statements should be understood as an aid to, rather than a substitute for, open dialogue between patients and health professionals.

Opportunistic or casual remarks by a healthy person reflecting distaste for life-prolonging treatment in the hypothetical event of incapacity are unlikely to meet the evidential requirements necessary to indicate an informed and considered decision. A general expression of views cannot be accorded the same weight as a firm decision. If representative of consistently manifested values, however, oral remarks contribute to the evaluation of the patient's interests. If witnessed and made by an informed individual, they could carry legal weight.

Many patients only lose capacity shortly before death. If suffering from illness requiring long-term in-patient or out-patient care, they have opportunities for discussion with the health-care team over a long period. They may feel their wishes are sufficiently well known or reflected in the notes so that there is no need to write them down. In hospice or specialist palliative care settings, this form of oral advance statement or directive (refusal) is common practice and appears to be respected.

In other situations, there is a risk that written advance statements might reduce rather than enhance the opportunities for discussion since inhibitions about raising the matter with health professionals lead some people to draft them in isolation. Individuals making an advance statement have to cope with difficult questions of their own mortality and loss of mental abilities as well as preparing for the fact that others may have to make crucial decisions of life and death for them. In such a situation, the patient will need counselling.

6.2 Written statements should use clear and unambiguous language. They should be signed by the individual and a witness. Model forms are available but clear statements in any format command respect.

There are no specific legal requirements concerning the format of the statement. The minimum requirements for the statement to be legally valid concern only the individual's competence, awareness of the implications of the decision and the relevance of the decision to the circumstances which arise (see Section 4).

It is clear that some people have a false impression that a written, witnessed statement carries more weight than their contemporaneous oral consent or refusal and so make statements for the wrong reasons. Health professionals must be aware of this and make all reasonable efforts to prevent such misunderstanding.

Health professionals can give advice that will lead to a well balanced declaration and they should be aware that their opinions and attitudes are likely to be influential even if they personally do not see the importance of writing an advance statement. They should record the patient's wishes about treatment and non-treatment in their own notes.

6.3 Patients have a legitimate expectation of being provided with information in an accessible form to allow them to make informed choices. Health professionals should ensure that the foreseeable options and implications are adequately explained, admit to uncertainty when this is the case and make reasonable efforts to discover if there is more specialised information available to pass on to the patient. An open attitude on the part of health professionals and a willingness to discuss the advantages and disadvantages of certain options can do much to establish trust and mutual understanding.

Foreseeable deterioration of mental faculties should be raised sensitively so that people can plan ahead without being pushed into committing themselves to a particular course. Any diagnosis of a life-threatening illness or deteriorating mental capacity must be backed by support and information so that patients can understand how their previous expectations for the future will be affected. The giving and receiving of bad news is likely to mark a new stage in the relationship between the patient and those providing health care. The existence of opportunities and receptiveness to discussion will affect how both sides experience the patient's illness. Insensitivity or lack of communication impacts on both. Good communication is not an optional extra service but an essential part of health care. It is important that health professionals have access to training in effective communication skills, and that there is a significant take-up of these opportunities.

GP practices may establish counselling and support sessions for people with conditions such as Alzheimer's disease. Funding may come from the GP's Health Promotion budget. Some surgeries and hospitals make available leaflets to help people consider treatment options in advance. People should be encouraged to take time to consider the issues carefully and ask questions. Routine consultation with the GP or practice nurse can provide such opportunities. Continuing specialist consultations, such as pain management clinics, also allow options to be discussed over a period of time.

6.4 Admittance to hospital, with its associated anxieties, is not generally a good time to raise the subject of anticipatory choice. Exceptions arise when the impetus for discussion comes from the patient or when sensitive discussion of cardiopulmonary resuscitation would be appropriate.

Admittance to hospital for treatment is stressful. Nevertheless, discussion of treatment options will sometimes arise then, either at the patient's initiation or because the patient's views need to be sought about cardiopulmonary resuscitation (CPR).

Discussion of resuscitation with all patients is inappropriate. The benefit and the patient's views may be beyond doubt, or there may be no expectation of CPR providing medical benefit. Sensitive exploration of the patient's wishes about CPR should be undertaken with patients who are at risk of cardiac or respiratory failure or who have a terminal illness. Ideally this should be done by the consultant. The views of the patient, where these can be ascertained, should be documented in the patient's records.

6.5 Advance statements should not he made under pressure. Professionals consulted at the drafting stage should take reasonable steps to ensure patients' decisions are not made under duress. Statements may evolve in stages over a period of time and discussion. It is inadvisable to conclude refusals or complicated statements in one discussion without further review. Patients should be reminded about the desirability of reviewing their statement on a regular basis, although a statement made long in advance is not automatically invalidated.

Time and support are required to come to terms with the full implications of bad news. Some people make clear that they do not want to know or else accept the knowledge in progressive stages. After considering the options, some patients will prefer decisions to be made for them by health professionals or other people they trust.

Health professionals and lawyers are often consulted at the time of drafting an advance statement. If in the course of discussing the statement they suspect there may be duress, they should take steps to counter it. This might, for example, take the form of arranging independent counselling for the patient.

Statements made long in advance of incapacity are not invalid but a regularly reviewed document is more likely to be applicable to the circumstances. Views change over time and, as the House of Lords Select Committee noted, 'disabled individuals are commonly more satisfied with their life than able-bodied people would expect to be with the same disability. The healthy do not choose in the same way as the sick'.[9]

6.6 Patients should be advised to avoid rushing into specifying future treatment when they have only recently received a prognosis or when they may be unduly influenced by others or when they are depressed.

6.7 Hospital managers and GP practice managers need to consider how to respond to the increasing desire by patients to plan ahead on the basis of accurate health information and advice.

There is no ideal moment to make an advance statement but there are clearly times which should be avoided. Health professionals providing information about prognosis or treatment options should advise patients of the risks of a premature or ill-considered decision.

Managers need to consider the provision of appropriately skilled staff, with time to discuss treatment implications. Giving bad news and helping patients make decisions on the basis of it is not a matter to be finalised on one occasion and adequate opportunities for discussion will need to be built into the health-care budget. Some hospitals retain specialised counsellors who provide information and support for in-patients and outpatients. With home visits they also have opportunities to discuss the options with other people who the patient wants to involve. Hospice outreach services and community nurses may also become involved in carrying out such a role. General practices and hospital policy makers will need to consider how to respond to patient demand for this type of service.

6.8 When responding to a request for assistance with advance statements, there are fundamental issues health professionals should consider:

- Does the patient have sufficient knowledge of the medical condition and possible treatment options if there is a known illness?
- Is the patient mentally competent?
- Is it clear that the patient is reflecting his or her own views and is not being pressured by other people?

Patients may have an unrealistic view of what medical science can or cannot do for them. Media reports sometimes result in an emotional declaration being written by people in a panic. There is a risk that such statements may take on a life of their own at a crucial moment without the writer having really foreseen the consequences. Impulsively written texts could be dangerous for the patient and confusing for the health team. Health professionals should attempt to give as much relevant factual information as possible in a form which the patient can assimilate. Often it will be difficult to avoid euphemisms and to give patients a clear view of the likely progression of the disease without also alarming or depressing them.

There are various opportunities for health professionals working in the community to discuss anticipatory decisions, such as when a person joins a GP practice or at times when regular health checks allow time for discussion with the doctor or practice nurse.

6.9 There are both advantages and disadvantages to making anticipatory decisions. Advance refusals are likely to be legally binding. Health professionals should try to ensure that patients are aware of drawbacks as well as advantages.

People are influenced by the type of advice and information they receive and how the options are portrayed to them. They need accurate information about the potential advantages and disadvantages of deciding in advance. Advance statements can have psychological and other benefits. Initiating discussion may clarify choices and enhance trust. Recording decisions gives a sense of control and peace of mind. Anecdotal reports recount cases of statements stored away by people who apparently made no effort to communicate their wishes; the discussion and drafting exercise apparently being sufficient. Statements can guide health professionals in difficult cases and remove the burden on people close to the patient.

The disadvantages include the risks of pressure or other forms of abuse and the impossibility of predicting how one might adapt to disabilities. Misdiagnosis might occur and unforeseen treatments may be developed. People might forget to amend the statement if their views change. Badly drafted statements can mislead or cause confusion and result in patients being treated differently than they intended or not treated at all.

7 Content of advance statements

7.1 Advance statements may list the individual's values as a basis for others to reach appropriate decisions. They may request all medically reasonable efforts be made to prolong life or express preferences between treatment options.

Advance statements can cover a range of matters, including both general views and specific decisions. Authorising statements (advance consent), although legally unenforceable, assist health professionals to accommodate decisions which are so personal that only the individual concerned could make them. A key concern for many people is to be able to say where they would like to be cared for and where they wish to die or who they want called to their bedside.

It is sometimes thought that clear and explicit advance refusals will most likely apply to futile treatments. Good professional practice should, in any event, ensure that these are not administered, and the courts have made clear that health professionals cannot be required to give treatment contrary to clinical judgement. Statements of advance consent are thus often seen as of more use and advance statements of views and preferences may be particularly helpful in non-emergency situations in determining what is in the patient's best interests.

7.2 Advance directives are specific refusals of treatment and can be legally binding (see Section 4).

7.3 Adults cannot authorise or refuse in advance, procedures which they could not authorise or refuse contemporaneously. They cannot authorise unlawful procedures or insist upon futile or inappropriate treatment.

As a matter of public policy, we have also stated that people should not be able to require withdrawal of basic care and comfort measures (see Section 5).

7.4 Women of childbearing age should be advised to consider the possibility of their advance statement or directive being invoked at a time when they are pregnant. A waiver covering pregnancy might be written into the statement.

7.5 If a patient is detained under the Mental Health Act, drugs with potentially damaging side effects may sometimes have to be prescribed without prior discussion with the patient. When the patient regains insight, advance statements about preferences between equally viable options for future treatment can be discussed and reflected in subsequent treatment plans.

Professionals providing mental health care have responsibilities for mentally disordered patients who may suffer recurrent psychotic episodes. If the patient has to be detained under the Mental Health Act, in some circumstances neuroleptics and other drugs (which may sometimes cause damaging side effects) may have to be prescribed without prior discussion with the patient. Once the patient recovers from a psychotic episode, health professionals have a key role in assisting the patient to evaluate and reconcile the advantages and disadvantages of the treatment and make decisions about future management accordingly. Anticipatory statements authorising treatment or expressing preferences between equally viable treatments can be discussed at times when the patient retains insight about the condition and these should be reflected in subsequent treatment plans. If, however, a patient is detained for compulsory treatment under Mental Health legislation, any advance refusal of treatment by the patient could be overruled (see Section 4).

8 Assessing mental capacity

8.1 Opportunities for assessing mental capacity arise at two points. First, an individual must have enough understanding of the implications in order to make a valid advance statement. Secondly, that statement will then speak for the patient at the point where he or she is considered to have insufficient understanding to make the particular decision in question.

Only when a person has or has had sufficient understanding and awareness to make a decision can significance attach to it. Capacity must always be assessed in relation to the decision in question. Health professionals are sometimes asked to make retrospective judgements about a patient's capacity. The BMA and the Law Society are producing detailed guidance for doctors and lawyers on this and other aspects of assessing capacity. A medical opinion about an individual's legal capacity may be open to challenge either by the person concerned or by another interested party.

8.2 When consulted by someone who wishes to draft an advance statement, health professionals should consider whether there are any reasons to doubt the patient's capacity to make the decisions in question. Capacity is assumed unless evidence suggests the contrary. The signature of a health professional as a witness may well imply that assessment of capacity has taken place.

The assessment of adult patients' capacities to make decisions about their own medical treatment is a matter for professional judgement guided by current practice and subject to legal requirements. Under normal circumstances, it is the personal responsibility of any health professional proposing to examine or to treat a patient to judge whether the patient has the capacity to give a valid consent. Similarly, if consulted to witness or assist in the drafting of an advance statement, health professionals should consider whether there are grounds for doubting the person's capacity and, if in doubt, seek a further opinion.

8.3 The High Court has held that a person has capacity if he or she can understand and retain the information relevant to the decision in question, can believe that information and can assess it in arriving at a choice.[10]

In order for an advance directive to be valid a patient must, at the time the statement was made, have had the capacity to understand and weigh the implications and consequences of that choice. The level of understanding required to make decisions must be commensurate with the gravity of the decision being made.

8.4 To demonstrate capacity individuals should be able to:

- Understand in broad terms and simple language what the medical treatment is, its purpose and nature and why it is or will be proposed for them
- Understand its principal benefits, risks and alternatives
- Understand in broad terms what will be the consequences of not receiving the proposed treatment
- Make a free choice (i.e. free from undue pressure)
- Retain the information long enough to make an effective decision.

It must be remembered that:

- There is a presumption of capacity until the contrary is demonstrated
- Any assessment of an individual's capacity has to be made in relation to a particular treatment proposal
- Capacity in an individual with a mental disorder can be variable over time and so health professionals should attempt to identify the time and manner most helpful to the patient when they might discuss the matter
- Capacity may be temporarily impaired due to toxic conditions or extreme illness
- All assessments of an individual's capacity should be fully recorded in the patient's medical, nursing and other appropriate notes.

9 Storage of advance statements

9.1 Storage of an advance statement and notification of its existence are primarily the responsibility of the individual. A copy of any written advance statement should be given to a person's general practitioner. People close to the patient should he made aware of the existence of an advance statement and be told where it is.

Some individuals carry a card, bracelet or other measure indicating the existence of an advance statement and where it is kept.

Once an advance statement has been made, it should be readily accessible when the need arises. It is the responsibility of the individual to ensure that his or her statement is available. General statements, made by healthy individuals, are best lodged with their general practitioner. This will allow the GP to provide the information to other health professionals on referral or, in emergency situations, to provide the information on request. For chronically ill patients, who are treated by a specialist team over a prolonged period, a copy of the advance statement should be in both relevant hospital files and the GP record.

9.2 For chronically ill patients, who are treated by a specialist team over a prolonged period, a copy of the advance statement should be in all relevant hospital files and the GP record.

Part IV – Implementation

10 General implementation

10.1 If health professionals know or have reasonable grounds to believe that an advance statement exists and time permits, they should make further enquiries. This could be by looking in relevant hospital notes, or contacting the general practitioner, or contacting people close to the patient.

Health professionals, once alerted to the existence of a relevant statement, should make reasonable efforts to find it. In an emergency where treatment delay might be fatal, clinical judgement must be exercised in deciding whether to follow the statement. When time permits, efforts must also be made to check the validity of any document presented. Basic verification includes checking that a written statement actually belongs to the patient who has been admitted, is dated, signed, preferably is witnessed and that there is no evidence to show it has been revoked.

10.2 Emergency treatment should not normally be delayed in order to look for an advance statement or refusal if there is no clear indication that one exists (see also Figure 2).

The principle of necessity allows health professionals to provide treatment (or to restrain medically or physically a person who may commit harm) without consent. The necessity justification applies mainly to emergency situations. Although the legal ground upon which such a justification is based is one of necessity, the language of consent may also be used. Consent in certain circumstances is 'implied' or 'presumed' or can be assumed will be obtained in the future.

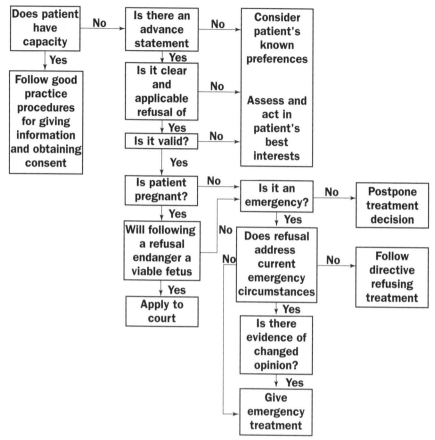

Figure 2 Implementing treatment flow chart

If a person is now incapacitated but is known to have objections to all or some treatment, health professionals may not be justified in proceeding, even in an emergency. They will need to consider the available evidence about the patient's views and how convincing it seems. A written, witnessed statement should be viewed as convincing unless contradictory evidence of a retraction is available. Previous oral statements refusing treatment may be valid but also require evaluation of the evidence. In the absence of evidence of refusal, treatment which is in the interests of that individual can be given.

If the incapacity is temporary because of anaesthetic, sedation, intoxication or temporary unconsciousness, health professionals should not proceed beyond what is essential to preserve the person's life or prevent deterioration in health. In other words, treatments which are 'necessary', in that it would generally be agreed to be unreasonable to postpone them, are to be distinguished from those which are merely convenient. Treatment which could reasonably be postponed until the patient regains competency should not be given.

10.3 In England, Wales and Northern Ireland, no-one is legally empowered to consent or refuse on behalf of an adult who lacks capacity to make the particular treatment decision.

10.4 In Scotland, some treatment decisions may be taken by a tutor dative. The views of people close to the patient can be helpful in identifying what he or she would want. Long-stay patients may also have discussed their wishes with nurses and other staff. When an adult lacks mental capacity to make or communicate the particular treatment decision, no other person is legally empowered to do so in England, Wales and Northern Ireland. Nor can competent people, facing mental incapacity, nominate others to make legally binding treatment choices for them.

In Scotland, the powers of a tutor dative might fulfil such a function. The authority of a tutor dative to refuse treatment on behalf of an incompetent patient would, it is thought, depend largely on whether the refusal conformed with the patient's own wishes and whether those could be shown to be informed and applicable. No case of refusal by a tutor dative has yet been heard in Scotland, but there may be little practical difference when compared with the position in England, Wales and Northern Ireland.

10.5 If an incapacitated pregnant woman presents with an apparently valid advance directive refusing treatment, legal advice should be sought to clarify the position.

If a mentally incapacitated and clearly pregnant woman presents with an apparently valid advance directive refusing treatment, legal advice should be sought. The courts may consider the advance refusal ineffective if withholding treatment endangers an otherwise viable fetus.

10.6 One type of particularly serious condition is the persistent vegetative state (pvs) where there is no chance of recovery, but where life is dependent on artificial feeding. Diagnosis of this condition can only be made after twelve months when it is due to head injury but six months if it is due to other causes. The courts have to be consulted before treatment can be withdrawn and so any directive relating to pvs should be put before the courts before it can take effect.

10.7 If doubt exists about what the individual intends, the law supports a presumption in favour of providing clinically appropriate treatment. Carers and nurses during their working relationship with long-stay patients in residential or in-patient settings, are likely to have an understanding of the patient's feelings and opinions. While these views should be taken into account they should not necessarily be determinative if in conflict with other evidence.

11 Liability of health professionals

11.1 Health professionals may be legally liable if they disregard the terms of an advance directive (i.e. refusal of treatment) if the directive is known of and applicable to the circumstances.

Health professionals following the terms of a clear advance directive (refusal of treatment) and exercising due care and attention would be very unlikely to face prosecution. The Crown Prosecution Service in its evidence to the House of Lords has endorsed the view that if an incompetent patient had previously made an advance directive (refusal), health professionals 'must abide by the terms of that previous expression of intention or wish, though special care may be necessary to ensure that any prior refusal of consent to medical treatment is still properly to be regarded as applicable in the circumstances which have subsequently occurred'.[11]

This Code provides, however, that an advance refusal of the minimally essential measures necessary to keep a patient comfortable ('basic care') should not be binding (see Section 5). In case of doubt, legal opinion should he sought. The Official Solicitor's office represents mentally incapacitated people's interests in legal matters and may be able to advise appropriate action, although a court ruling or declaratory judgement may

149

be required. Health professionals must always act with due care and attention. For example, the mistaken application of an advance refusal to a patient other than the one who made it may raise issues of negligence.

11.1.1 Applicability: If the situation is not identical to that described in the advance statement or refusal, it is still advisable to act in the general spirit of the statement, if this is clearly described. If any individuals are named in the statement for contact, they, as well as the GP may be able to clarify the patient's wishes. If there is doubt, however, as to what a patient intended, the law supports a presumption that appropriate life-prolonging measures should be given. Health professionals must use their own professional judgement about the appropriateness of the statement. If a refusal is not applicable to the circumstances, it is not legally binding although it may still give valuable indications of the general treatment options the patient would prefer. If a statement requests or consents to certain options, for example, the health team will have to judge whether the treatment is medically appropriate or advisable for that patient at that time.

12 Disputes

12.1 In the event of disagreement between health professionals or between health professionals and people close to the patient, the senior clinician must consider the available evidence of the patient's wishes.

Junior medical and other staff should ensure that the senior professional managing the case is kept aware of the patient's oral wishes or written statement. There may, however, be clinical reasons for not complying with a patient's requests or preferences. A clear, applicable advance refusal will have legal force and the consultant should be informed of this. Thereafter, junior medical, nursing and other professional staff should accept the judgement of the clinician in overall charge of the patient.

12.2 In cases of doubt or disagreement about the scope or validity of an advance directive (refusal), emergency treatment should normally be given and advice sought from the courts if the matter cannot be clarified in any other way.

In the event of disagreement between health professionals or between relatives and health professionals about the patient's previously expressed wishes, opinions should be sought from relevant colleagues and others who are familiar with the patient. The point of discussion should not be to override the patient's view but to clarify its scope and seek evidence concerning its validity. Ultimately, the senior professional managing the particular episode of the patient's care should take responsibility and may need to seek advice from the courts if the matter cannot be clarified.

12.3 In any case of dispute, legal judgement will be based upon the strength of the evidence. Disagreements may arise between a hospital doctor and a GP or between nursing and medical staff in a hospital. All staff involved in a patient's care should have an opportunity of presenting their views. From a patient's viewpoint, nurses are often the most accessible professional. Hospital or community nurses may, over a period of time, have had closer contact than others with the patient and with those close to the patient. Nurses are often adept in translating technical medical language and discussing practical aspects of outcomes of treatment and care. They may gain particular insight into whether patients were consistent and coherent in their views.

13 *Conscientious objection*

13.1 Some health professionals disagree in principle with patients' rights to refuse life-prolonging treatment but may nonetheless support advance statements which express preferences.

13.2 Health professionals are entitled to have their personal moral beliefs respected and not be pressurised to act contrary to those beliefs. But the 'sanctity of life' argument or other values must not be imposed upon those for whom they have or had no meaning.

13.3 Health professionals with a conscientious objection to limiting treatment at a patient's request should make their view clear when the patient initially raises the matter. In such cases the patient should he advised of the option of seeing another health professional if the patient wishes.

13.4 If a health professional is involved in the management of a case and cannot for reasons of conscience accede to a patient's request for limitation of treatment, management of that patient must be passed to a colleague.

13.5 In an emergency, if no other health professional is available there is a legal duty to comply with an appropriate and valid advance refusal. Some doctors and nurses have moral objections to withholding life-prolonging treatment. Their views should be respected and they must not be marginalised within the health care service. The people they care for have the right to know as far as possible how their requests or refusals will be received. Health professionals with a conscientious objection should make that clear when the patient initially raises the matter so that the patient can decide how to proceed. Health professionals unable to limit treatment on request should step aside and pass management of that patient to a colleague. In an emergency, if delegation is impossible, the doctor or nurse must comply with a valid advance directive (treatment refusal). It is unacceptable to force treatment upon a patient.

PART V – Summary

14 Summary

14.1 Although not binding on health professionals, advance statements deserve thorough consideration and respect.

14.2 Where valid and applicable, advance directives (refusals) must be followed.

14.3 Health professionals consulted by people wishing to formulate an advance statement or directive should take all reasonable steps to provide accurate factual information about the treatment options and their implications.

14.4 Where an unknown and incapacitated patient presents for treatment some checks should be made concerning the validity of any directive refusing life-prolonging treatment. In all cases, it is vital to check that the statement or refusal presented is that of the patient being treated and has not been withdrawn.

14.5 If the situation is not identical to that described in the advance statement or refusal, treatment providers may still be guided by the general spirit of the statement if this is evident. it is advisable to contact any person nominated by the patient as well as the GP to clarify the patient's wishes. If there is doubt as to what the patient intended, the law requires the exercise of a best interests judgement.

14.6 If an incapacitated person is known to have had sustained and informed objections to all or some treatment, even though these have not been formally recorded, health professionals may not be justified in proceeding. This applies even in an emergency.

If witnessed and made at a time when the patient was competent and informed, such objections may constitute an oral advance directive. Health professionals will need to consider how much evidence is available about the patient's decisions and how convincing it seems. All members of the health care team can make a useful contribution to this process.

14.7 In the absence of any indication of the patient's wishes, there is a common law duty to give appropriate treatment to incapacitated patients when the treatment is clearly in their best interests.

Checklist for writing an advance statement

In drawing up an advance statement you must ensure, as a minimum, that the following information is included:

- Full name
- Address
- Name and address of general practitioner
- Whether advice was sought from health professionals
- Signature
- Date drafted and reviewed
- Witness signature
- A clear statement of your wishes, either general or specific
- The name, address and telephone number of your nominated person, if you have one.

References

1 *Re C [Adult: Refusal of Medical Treatment]* (1994) 1 WLR 290.
2 *per* Lord Templeton in *Sidaway v. Board of Governors of the Bethlem Royal Hospital and Maudsley Hospital* (1985) AC 871.
3 *Re T [Adult: Refusal of Treatment]* (1993) Fam 95.
4 Lord Donaldson in *Re T [Adult: Refusal of Treatment]* (1993) Fam 95, 5.
5 *Airedale NHS Trust v. Bland* (1993) AC 789.
6 *Re C [Adult: Refusal of Medical Treatment]* (1994) 1 WLR 290.
7 See para 2.6 of *Mental Health Act Code of Practice*, HMSO, August 1993 (England and Wales). Similar Codes of Practice have also been issued for Scotland (Mental Health Act: Code of Practice (Scotland)) and for Northern Ireland (Code of Practice for Mental Health Orders (N. Ireland)).
8 See para 2.6 of *Mental Health Act Code of Practice*, HMSO, August 1993 (England and Wales). Similar Codes of Practice have also been issued for Scotland (Mental Health Act: Code of Practice (Scotland)) and for Northern Ireland (Code of Practice for Mental Health Orders (N. Ireland)).
9 *Report from the Select Committee on Medical Ethics*, HMSO, 1994, Vol 1, p.41. A new stage in a patient's illness may be an appropriate time to review earlier stated wishes. Computerised annual recall facilities may be a way for GPs to remind patients to review their advance statements.
10 *Re C [Adult: Refusal of Medical Treatment]* (1994) 1 WLR 290.
11 *Report from the Select Committee on Medical Ethics*, HMSO, 1994, Vol 1, p.39.

Appendix II:
Shape your health care future with Health Care Advance Directives

Caution: This booklet presents general information about the law and does not necessary apply to your individual situation or constitute legal advice. Every person's circumstances are different. Also, laws vary from state to state [as well as from country to country] … Therefore, it is important to seek advice about your own state's law and how it applies to your situation.

This publication was produced and funded by the American Association of Retired Persons, the American Bar Association Commission on Legal Problems of the Elderly, and the American Medical Association.

What is a Health Care Advance Directive?

A Health Care Advance Directive is a document in which you give instructions about your health care if, in the future, you cannot speak for yourself. You can give someone you name (your 'agent' or 'proxy') the power to make health care decisions for you. You also can give instructions about the kind of health care you do or do not want.

In a traditional Living Will, you state your wishes about life-sustaining medical treatments if you are terminally ill. In a Health Care Power of Attorney, you appoint someone else to make medical treatment decisions for you if you cannot make them for yourself.

The Health Care Advance Directive in this booklet combines and expands the traditional Living Will and Health Care Power of Attorney into a single, comprehensive document.

Why is it useful?

Unlike most Living Wills, a Health Care Advance Directive is not limited to cases of terminal illness. If you cannot make or communicate decisions because of a temporary or permanent illness or injury, a Health Care Advance Directive helps you keep control over health care decisions that are important to you. In your Health Care Advance Directive, you state your wishes about any aspect of your health care, including decisions about life-sustaining treatment, and choose a person to make and communicate these decisions for you.

Appointing an agent is particularly important. At the time a decision needs to be made, your agent can participate in discussions and weigh the pros and cons of treatment decisions based on your wishes. Your agent can decide for you wherever you cannot decide for yourself, even if your decision-making ability is only temporarily affected.

Unless you formally appoint someone to decide for you, many health care providers and institutions will make critical decisions for you that might not be based on your wishes. In some situations, a court may have to appoint a guardian unless you have an advance directive.

An advance directive also can relieve family stress. By expressing your wishes in advance, you help family or friends who might otherwise struggle to decide on their own what you would want done.

Are Health Care Advance Directives legally valid in every state?

Yes. Every state and the District of Columbia has laws that permit individuals to sign documents stating their wishes about health care decisions when they cannot speak for themselves. The specifics of these laws vary, but the basic principle of listening to the patient's wishes is the same everywhere. The law gives great weight to any form of written directive. If the courts become involved, they usually try to follow the patient's stated values and preferences, especially if they are in written form. A Health Care Advance Directive may be the most convincing evidence of your wishes you can create.

What does a Health Care Advance Directive say?

There are two parts to the Health Care Advance Directive in this booklet.

The most important part of the advance directive is the appointment of someone (your agent) to make health care decisions for you if you cannot decide for yourself. You can define how much or how little authority you want your agent to have. You also can name persons to act as alternate agents if your primary agent cannot act for you, and disqualify specific persons whom you do not want to make decisions for you.

If there is no one whom you trust fully to serve as your agent, then you should not name an agent. Instead, you can rely on the second part of the Advance Directive to make your wishes known.

In the second part of the Advance Directive, you can provide specific instructions about your health care treatment. You also can include a statement about donating your organs. Your instructions in the second part provide evidence of your wishes that your agent, or anyone providing you with medical care, should follow.

You can complete either or both parts of the Health Care Advance Directive.

How do I make a Health Care Advance Directive?

The process for creating a Health Care Advance Directive depends on where you live. Most states have laws that provide special forms and signing procedures.

Most states also have special witnessing requirements and restrictions on whom you can appoint as your agent (such as prohibiting a health care provider from being your agent). Follow these rules carefully.

Typically, states require two witnesses. Some require or permit a notarized signature. Some have special witnessing requirements if you live in a nursing home or similar facility. Even where witnesses are not required, consider using them anyway to reinforce the deliberate nature of your act and to increase the likelihood that care providers in other states will accept the document.

If you use the form included here, you should be able to meet most states' requirements. However, you may want to check the rules in your state.

If I change my mind, can I cancel or change a Health Care Advance Directive?

Yes, you can cancel or change your Health Care Advance Directive by telling your agent or health care provider in writing of your decision to do so. Destroying all copies of the old one and creating a new one is the best way. Make sure you give a copy of the new one to your physician and anyone else who received the old one.

What do I need to consider before making a Health Care Advance Directive?

There are at least four important questions to ask yourself:

First – What are my goals for medical treatment? The Health Care Advance Directive may determine what happens to you over a period of disability or at the very final stage of your life. You can help others respect your wishes if you take some steps now to make your treatment preferences clear.

While it is impossible to anticipate all of the different medical decisions that may come up, you can make your preferences clear by stating your goals for medical treatment. What do you want treatment to accomplish? Is it enough that treatment could prolong your life, whatever your quality of life? Or, if life-sustaining treatment could not restore consciousness or your ability to communicate with family members or friends, would you rather stop treatment?

Once you have stated your goals of treatment, your family and physicians can make medical decisions for you on the basis of your goals. If treatment would help achieve one of your goals, the treatment would be provided. If treatment would not help achieve one of your goals, the treatment would not be provided.

In formulating your goals of treatment, it is often helpful to consider your wishes about different end-of-life treatments and then asking yourself why do you feel that way. If you would not want to be kept alive by a ventilator, what is it about being on a ventilator that troubles you? Is it the loss of mobility, the lack of independence, or some other factor? Would it matter if you needed a ventilator for only a few days rather than many months? The answers to these kinds of questions will reflect important values that you hold and that will help you shape your goals of treatment.

Another way to become clear about your goals of treatment is to create a 'Values History.' In doing a Values History, you examine your values and attitudes, discuss them with loved ones or advisers and write down your responses to questions such as:

- How do you feel about your current health?
- How important is independence and self-sufficiency in your life?
- How do you imagine handling illness, disability, dying, and death?
- How might your personal relationships affect medical decision-making, especially near the end of life?
- What role should doctors and other health professionals play in such decisions?
- What kind of living environment is important to you if you become seriously ill or disabled?
- How much should the cost to your family be a part of the decision-making process?
- What role do religious beliefs play in decisions about your health care?
- What are your thoughts about life in general in its final stages: your hopes and fears, enjoyments and sorrows?

Once you have identified your values, you can use them to decide what you want medical treatment to accomplish.

Second – Who should be my agent? Choosing your agent is the most important part of this process. Your agent will have great power over your health and personal care if you cannot make your own decisions. Normally, no one oversees or monitors your agent's decisions.

Choose one person to serve as your agent to avoid disagreements. If you appoint two or more agents to serve together and they disagree, your medical caregivers will have no clear direction. If possible, appoint at least one alternate agent in case your primary agent is not available.

Speak to the person (and alternate agents) you wish to appoint before-hand to explain your desires. Confirm their willingness to act for you and their understanding of your wishes. Also be aware that some states will not let certain persons (such as your doctor) act as your agent. If you can think of no one you trust to carry out this responsibility, then do not name an agent. Make sure, however, that you provide instructions that will guide your doctor or a court-appointed decision-maker.

Third – How specific should I be? A Health Care Advance Directive does not have to give directions or guidelines for your agent. However, if you have specific wishes or preferences, it is important to spell them out in the document itself. Also discuss them with your agent and health care providers. These discussions will help ensure that your wishes, values and preferences will be respected. Make sure to think about your wishes about artificial feeding (nutrition and hydration), since people sometimes have very different views on this topic.

At the same time, be aware that you cannot cover all the bases. It is impossible to predict all the circumstances you may face. Simple statements like 'I never want to be placed on a ventilator' may not reflect your true wishes. You might want ventilator assistance if it were temporary and you then could resume your normal activities. No matter how much direction you provide, your agent will still need considerable discretion and flexibility. Write instructions carefully so they do not restrict the authority of your agent in ways you did not intend.

Fourth – How can I make sure that health care providers will follow my Advance Directive? Regardless of the laws about advance directives in your state, some physicians, hospitals or other health care providers may have personal views or values that do not agree with your stated desires. As a result, they may not want to follow your Health Care Advance Directive.

Most state laws give doctors the right to refuse to honor your advance directive on conscience grounds. However, they generally must help you find a doctor or hospital that will honor your directive. The best way to avoid this problem is to talk to your physician and other health care providers ahead of time. Make sure they understand the document and your wishes, and they have no objections. If there are objections, work them out, or change physicians.

Once you sign a Health Care Advance Directive, be sure to give a copy of it to your doctor and to your agent, close relatives, and anyone else who may be involved in your care.

What happens if I do not have an Advance Directive?

If you do not have an Advance Directive and you cannot make health care decisions, some state laws give decision-making power to default decision-makers or 'surrogates'. These surrogates, who are usually family members in order of kinship, can make some or all health care decisions. Some states authorize a 'close friend' to make decisions, but usually only when family members are unavailable.

Even without such statutes, most doctors and health facilities routinely consult family, as long as there are close family members available and there is no disagreement. However, problems can arise because family members may not know what the patient would want in a given situation. They also may disagree about the best course of action. Disagreement can easily undermine family consent. A hospital physician or specialist who does not know you well may become your decision-maker, or a court proceeding may be necessary to resolve a disagreement.

In these situations, decisions about your health care may not reflect your wishes or may be made by persons you would not choose. Family members and persons close to you may go through needless agony in making life and death decisions without your guidance. It is far better to make your wishes known and appoint an agent ahead of time through a Health Care Advance Directive.

Who can help me create a Health Care Advance Directive?

You do not need a lawyer to make a Health Care Advance Directive. However, a lawyer can be helpful if your family situation is uncertain or complex, or you expect problems to arise. Start by talking to someone who knows you well and can help you state your values and wishes considering your family and medical history.

Your doctor is an important participant in creating your Health Care Advance Directive. Discuss the kinds of medical problems you may face, based on your current health and health history. Your doctor can help you understand the treatment choices your agent may face. Share your ideas for instructions with your doctor to make sure medical care providers can understand them.

You can obtain up-to-date, state-by-state information about Advance Directives, along with statutory forms, if they exist in your state, from:

Legal Counsel for the Elderly (LCE)
American Association of Retired Persons
P.O. Box 96474
Washington, DC 20090-6474.

LCE has state-specific guidebooks about advance directives. If you want to order a booklet, send $5 per booklet (for shipping and handling) to the above address.

Choice In Dying, Inc., a non-profit educational organization located at 200 Varick Street, New York, NY 10014-4810. Telephone: 1-800-989-WILL.

Hospital associations, medical societies or bar associations in your state or county, or your local area agency on aging (AAA) may provide forms for your state.

If your state has a statutory form, remember that preprinted forms – including the one contained in this booklet – may not meet all your needs. Take the time to consider all possibilities and seek advice so that the document you develop meets your special needs.

If you want legal help, contact your state or local Office on Aging. These offices usually are quite familiar with health care issues and local resources for legal assistance. You also can contact the bar association for your state or locality. Its lawyer referral service may be able to refer you to an attorney who handles this type of matter. Finally, organizations that deal with planning for incapacity, such as your local Alzheimer's Association chapter, may be able to provide advice or referrals.

Health Care Advance Directive

Form and instructions

Caution: This Health Care Advance Directive is a general form provided for your convenience. While it meets the legal requirements of most states, it may or may not fit the requirements of your particular state. Many states have special forms or special procedures for creating Health Care Advance Directives. Even if your state's law does not clearly recognize this document, it may still provide an effective statement of your wishes if you cannot speak for yourself.

Section 1 – Health care agent

Print your full name here as the 'principal' or creator of the health care advance directive.

Print the full name, address and telephone number of the person (age 18 or older) you appoint as your health care agent. Appoint only a person with whom you have talked and whom you trust to understand and carry out your values and wishes.

Many states limit the persons who can serve as your agent. If you want to meet all existing state restrictions do not name any of the following as your agent, since some states will not let them act in that role:

- your health care providers, including physicians;

- staff of health care facilities or nursing care facilities providing your care;

- guardians of your finances (also called conservators);

- employees of government agencies financially responsible for your care;

- any person serving as agent for 10 or more persons.

Section 2 – Alternate agents

It is a good idea to name alternate agents in case your first agent is not available. Of course, only appoint alternates if you fully trust them to act faithfully as your agent and you have talked to them about serving as your agent. Print the appropriate information in this paragraph. You can name as many alternate agents as you wish, but place them in the order you wish them to serve.

Section 3 – Effective date and durability

This sample document is effective if and when you cannot make health care decisions. Your agent and your doctor determine if you are in this condition. Some state laws include specific procedures for determining your decision-making ability. If you wish, you can include other effective dates or other criteria for determining that you cannot make health care decisions (such as requiring two physicians to evaluate your decision-making ability). You also can state that the power will end at some later date or event before death.

In any case, you have the right to revoke or take away the agent's authority at any time. To revoke, notify your agent or health care provider orally or in writing. If you revoke, it is best to notify in writing both your agent and physician and anyone else who has a copy of the directive. Also destroy the health care advance directive document itself.

Health Care Advance Directive Part I: Appointment of health care agent

1 Health care agent

I, _____

hereby appoint:

Agent's name _____

Address _____

_____

_____

Home phone no. _____

Work phone no. _____

as my agent to make health and personal care decisions for me as authorized in this document.

2 Alternate agents

- If I revoke my agent's authority; or

- If my agent becomes unwilling or unavailable to act; or

- If my agent is my spouse and I become legally separated or divorced;

I name the following (each to act alone and successively, in the order named) as alternates to my agent.

A. First Alternate Agent

_____

Address _____

_____

_____

Telephone _____

B. Second Alternate Agent

_____

Address _____

_____

_____

Telephone _____

3 Effective date and durability

By this document I intend to create a Health Care Advance Directive. It is effective upon, and only during, any period in which I cannot make or communicate a choice regarding a particular health care decision. My agent, attending physician and any other necessary experts should determine that I am unable to make choices about health care.

Section 4 – Agent's powers

This grant of power is intended to be as broad as possible. Unless you set limits, your agent will have authority to make any decision you could make to obtain or stop any type of health care.

Even under this broad grant of authority, your agent still must follow your wishes and directions, communicated by you in any manner now or in the future.

To specifically limit or direct your agent's power, you must complete Section 6 in Part II of the advance directive.

4 Agent's powers

I give my agent full authority to make health care decisions for me. My agent shall follow my wishes as known to my agent either through this document or through other means. When my agent interprets my wishes, I intend my agent's authority to be as broad as possible, except for any limitations I state in this form. In making any decision, my agent shall try to discuss the proposed decision with me to determine my desires if I am able to communicate in any way. If my agent cannot determine the choice I would want, then my agent shall make a choice for me based upon what my agent believes to be in my best interests.

Unless specifically limited by Section 6, below, my agent is authorized as follows:

A To consent, refuse, or withdraw consent to any and all types of health care. Health care means any care, treatment, service or procedure to maintain, diagnose or otherwise affect an individual's physical or mental condition. It includes, but is not limited to, artificial respiration, nutritional support and hydration, medication and cardiopulmonary resuscitation;

B To have access to medical records and information to the same extent that I am entitled, including the right to disclose the contents to others as appropriate for my health care;

C To authorize my admission to or discharge (even against medical advice) from any hospital, nursing home, residential care, assisted living or similar facility or service;

D To contract on my behalf for any health care related service or facility on my behalf, without my agent incurring personal financial liability for such contracts;

E To hire and fire medical, social service, and other support personnel responsible for my care;

F To authorize, or refuse to authorize, any medication or procedure intended to relieve pain, even though such use may lead to physical damage, addiction, or hasten the moment of (but not intentionally cause) my death;

G To make anatomical gifts of part or all of my body for medical purposes, authorize an autopsy, and direct the disposition of my remains, to the extent permitted by law;

H To take any other action necessary to do what I authorize here, including (but not limited to) granting any waiver or release from liability required by any hospital, physician, or other health care provider; signing any documents relating to refusals of treatment or the leaving of a facility against medical advice; and pursuing any legal action in my name at the expense of my estate to force compliance with my wishes as determined by my agent, or to seek actual or punitive damages for the failure to comply.

Section 5 – My instructions about end-of-life treatment

The subject of end-of-life treatment is particularly important to many people. In this paragraph, you can give general or specific instructions on the subject. The different paragraphs are options – choose only one, or write your desires or instructions in your own words (in the last option). If you are satisfied with your agent's knowledge of your values and wishes and you do not want to include instructions in the form, initial the first option and do not give instructions in the form.

Any instructions you give here will guide your agent. If you do not appoint an agent, they will guide any health care provider or surrogate decision-makers who must make a decision for you if you cannot do so yourself. The instruction choices in the form describe different treatment goals you may prefer, depending on your condition.

Directive in your own words

If you would like to state your wishes about end-of-life treatment in your own words instead of choosing one of the options provided, you can do so in this section. Since people sometimes have different opinions on whether nutrition and hydration should be refused or stopped under certain circumstances, be sure to address this issue clearly in your directive. Nutrition and hydration means food and fluids given through a nasogastric tube or tube into your stomach, intestines, or veins, and does not include non-intrusive methods such as spoon feeding or moistening of lips and mouth.

Some states allow the stopping of nutrition and hydration only if you expressly authorize it. If you are creating your own directive, and you do not want nutrition and hydration, state so clearly.

Health Care Advance Directive Part II: Instructions about health care

5 My instructions about end-of life treatment

(Initial only ONE of the following statements)

☐ No specific instructions. My agent knows my values and wishes, so I do not wish to include any specific instructions here.

☐ Directive to withhold or withdraw treatment. Although I greatly value life, I also believe that at some point, life has such diminished value that medical treatment should be stopped, and I should be allowed to die. Therefore, I do not want to receive treatment, including nutrition and hydration, when the treatment will not give me a meaningful quality of life. I do not want my life prolonged:

- If the treatment will leave me in a condition of permanent unconsciousness, such as with an irreversible coma or a persistent vegetative state

- If the treatment will leave me with no more than some consciousness and in an irreversible condition of complete, or nearly complete, loss of ability to think or communicate with others

- If the treatment will leave me with no more than some ability to think or communicate with others, and the likely risks and burdens of treatment outweigh the expected benefits. Risks, burdens and benefits include consideration of length of life, quality of life, financial costs, and my personal dignity and privacy.

Directive to receive treatment

I want my life to be prolonged as long as possible, no matter what my quality of life.

Directive about end-of-life treatment in my own words:

_____

_____

_____

_____

Section 6 – Any other health care instructions or limitations or modifications of my agent's powers

In this section, you can provide instructions about other health care issues that are not end-of-life treatment or nutrition and hydration. For example, you might want to include your wishes about issues like non-emergency surgery, elective medical treatments or admission to a nursing home. Again, be careful in these instructions not to place limitations on your agent that you do not intend. For example, while you may not want to be admitted to a nursing home, placing such a restriction may make things impossible for your agent if other options are not available.

You also may limit your agent's powers in any way you wish. For example, you can instruct your agent to refuse any specific types of treatment that are against your religious beliefs or unacceptable to you for any other reasons. These might include blood transfusions, electro-convulsive therapy, sterilization, abortion, amputation, psychosurgery, or admission to a mental institution, etc. Some states limit your agent's authority to consent to or refuse some of these procedures, regardless of your health care advance directive.

Be very careful about stating limitations, because the specific circumstances surrounding future health care decisions are impossible to predict. If you do not want any limitations, simply write in "No limitations".

Section 7 – Protection of third parties who rely on my agent

In most states, health care providers cannot be forced to follow the directions of your agent if they object. However most states also require providers to help transfer you to another provider who is willing to honor your instructions. To encourage compliance with the health care advance directive, this paragraph states that providers who rely in good faith on the agent's statements and decisions will not be held civilly liable for their actions.

Section 8 – Donation of organs at death

In this section you can state your intention to donate bodily organs and tissues at death. If you do not wish to be an organ donor, initial the first option. The second option is a donation of any or all organs or parts. The third option allows you to donate only those organs or tissues you specify. Consider mentioning the heart, liver, lung, kidney, pancreas, intestine, cornea, bone, skin, heart valves, tendons, ligaments, and saphenous vein in the leg. Finally, you may limit the use of your organs by crossing out any of the four purposes listed that you do not want (transplant, therapy, research or education). If you do not cross out any of these options, your organs may be used for any of these purposes.

6 Any other health care instructions or limitations or modifications of my agent's powers

_____

_____

_____

_____

7 Protection of third parties who rely on my agent

No person who relies in good faith upon any representations by my agent or alternate agent(s) shall be liable to me, my estate, my heirs or assigns, for recognizing the agent's authority.

Upon my death (initial one):

☐ I do not wish to donate any organs or tissue, OR

☐ I give any needed organs, tissues, or parts, OR

☐ I give only the following organs, tissues, or parts (please specify):

_____

_____

My gift (if any) is for the following purposes (cross out any of the following you do not want):

- Transplant

- Research

- Therapy

- Education

Section 9 – Nomination of guardian

Appointing a health care agent helps to avoid a court-appointed guardian for health care decision-making. However, if a court becomes involved for any reason, this paragraph expressly names your agent to serve as guardian. A court does not have to follow your nomination, but normally it will honor your wishes unless there is good reason to override your choice.

Section 10 – Administrative provisions

These items address miscellaneous matters that could affect the implementation of your Health Care Advance Directive.

Signing the document

Required state procedures for signing this kind of document vary. Some require only a signature, while others have very detailed witnessing requirements. Some states simply require notarization.

The procedure in this booklet is likely to be far more complex than your state law requires because it combines the formal requirements from virtually every state. Follow it if you do not know your state's requirements and you want to meet the signature requirements of virtually every state.

First, sign and date the document in the presence of two witnesses and a notary.

Nomination of guardian

If a guardian of my person should for any reason need to be appointed, I nominate my agent (or his or her alternate then authorized to act), named above.

Administrative provisions

(All apply)

- I revoke any prior health care advance directive.
- This health care advance directive is intended to be valid in any jurisdiction in which it is presented.
- A copy of this advance directive is intended to have the same effect as the original.

Signing the document

By signing here I indicate that I understand the contents of this document and the effect of this grant of powers to my agent.

I sign my name to this Health Care Advance Directive on this _____ day of _____ 20____

My signature _____

My name _____

My current home address is _____

_____

_____

Your witnesses should know your identity personally and be able to declare that you appear to be of sound mind and under no duress or undue influence.

In order to meet the different witnessing requirements of most states, do not have the following people witness your signature:

● Anyone you have chosen to make health care decisions on your behalf (agent or alternate agents).

● Your treating physician, health care provider, health facility operator, or an employee of any of these.

● Insurers or employees of your life/health insurance provider.

● Anyone financially responsible for your health care costs.

● Anyone related to you by blood, marriage, or adoption.

● Anyone entitled to any part of your estate under an existing will or by operation of law, or anyone who will benefit financially from your death. Your creditors should not serve as witnesses.

If you are in a nursing home or other institution, a few states have additional witnessing requirements. This form does not include witnessing language for this situation. Contact a patient advocate or an ombudsman to find out about the state's requirements in these cases.

Second, have your signature notarized. Some states permit notarization as an alternative to witnessing. Doing both witnessing and notarization is more than most states require, but doing both will meet the execution requirements of most states.

This form includes a typical notary statement, but it is wise to check state law in case it requires a special form of notary acknowledgment.

Witness statement

I declare that the person who signed or acknowledged this document is personally known to me, that he/she signed or acknowledged this health care advance directive in my presence, and that he/she appears to be of sound mind and under no duress, fraud, or undue influence.

I am not:

- The person appointed as agent by this document,
- The principal's health care provider,
- An employee of the principal's health care provider,
- Financially responsible for the principal's health care,
- Related to the principal by blood, marriage, or adoption, and,
- To the best of my knowledge, a creditor of the principal/or entitled to any part of his/her estate under a will now existing or by operation of law.

Witness no. 1

Signature _____

Date _____

Print Name _____

Telephone_____

Residence Address _____

_____

_____

Witness no. 2

Signature _____

Date _____

Print Name _____

Telephone _____

Residence Address _____

_____

_____

Notarization

State of _____

County of _____

On this _____ day of _____ 20____

The said _____,

known to me (or satisfactorily proven) to be the person named in the foregoing instrument personally appeared before me, a Notary Public, within and for the State and County aforesaid, and acknowledged that he or she freely and voluntarily executed the same for the purposes stated therein.

My Commission Expires: _____

Notary Public

Useful addresses

Alzheimer's Society
Gordon House
10 Greencoat Place
London SW1P 1PH
Tel: 020 7306 0606

Motor Neurone Disease Association
PO Box 246
Northampton NN1 2PR
Tel: 01604 250505
Helpline: 08457 626262

Patients' Association
PO Box 935
Harrow
Middlesex HA1 3YJ
Tel: 020 8423 8999

Terrence Higgins Trust and Kings College London
52–54 Grays Inn Road
London WC1X 8JU
Tel: 020 7831 0330
For people who are HIV positive

Voluntary Euthanasia Society
13 Prince of Wales Terrace
London W8 5PG
Tel: 020 7937 7770

About Age Concern

Their Rights: advance directives and living wills explored is one of a wide range of publications produced by Age Concern England, the National Council on Ageing. Age Concern works on behalf of all older people and believes later life should be fulfilling and enjoyable. For too many this is impossible. As the leading charitable movement in the UK concerned with ageing and older people, Age Concern finds effective ways to change that situation.

Where possible, we enable older people to solve problems themselves, providing as much or as little support as they need. A network of local Age Concerns, supported by 250,000 volunteers, provides community-based services such as lunch clubs, day centres and home visiting.

Nationally, we take a lead role in campaigning, parliamentary work, policy analysis, research, specialist information and advice provision, and publishing. Innovative programmes promote healthier lifestyles and provide older people with opportunities to give the experience of a lifetime back to their communities.

Age Concern is dependent on donations, covenants and legacies.

Age Concern England
1268 London Road
London SW16 4ER
Tel: 020 8765 7200
Fax: 020 8765 7211

Age Concern Cymru
4th Floor
1 Cathedral Road
Cardiff CF1 9SD
Tel: 029 2037 1566
Fax: 029 2039 9562

Age Concern Scotland
113 Rose Street
Edinburgh EH2 3DT
Tel: 0131 220 3345
Fax: 0131 220 2779

Age Concern Northern Ireland
3 Lower Crescent
Belfast BT7 1NR
Tel: 028 9024 5729
Fax: 028 9023 5497

Publications from Age Concern Books

Residents' Money: A guide to good practice in care homes

Residents' Money is a guide for people who work in residential and nursing homes who may be involved in handling residents' money or in helping them to manage their financial affairs. It includes detailed advice for care managers and staff on how to design and put into practice policies that reflect the very best in good practice.

£7.99 0-86242-205-1

Managing Other People's Money, 2nd Edition

Penny Letts

Ideal for both the family carer and for legal and other advice workers. *Managing Other People's Money* is essential reading for anyone facing this challenging situation. Providing a step-by-step guide to the arrangements which have to be made, topics include:

- when to take over
- the powers available
- enduring power of attorney
- Court of Protection
- claiming benefits
- collecting pensions and salaries
- living arrangements
- residential care.

£9.99 0-86242-250-7

(Please note this book does not cover legal arrangements in Scotland or Northern Ireland)

Promoting Mobility for People with Dementia: A problem-solving approach

Rosemary Oddy

People with dementia must be enabled to move and given the opportunity to do so frequently, with or without help, if they are to remain mobile. The common sense approaches described in this book should ease the task of retaining optimum levels of mobility for people with dementia for as long as possible, without jeopardising the health and safety of those who care for them. With the wealth of ideas contained in this book, physiotherapists, occupational therapists, nurses and carers will find plenty to stimulate the imagination.

£14.99 0-86242-242-6

Money at Home: The home care worker's guide to handling other people's finances

Pauline Thompson

Whenever money is handled for a service user, the home care worker is placed in a position of trust, even if it is just a one-off occasion. In the vast majority of cases, there are no problems but, even in the best relationships, misunderstandings can occur or the unexpected happen. This guide covers some of the key issues to consider in handling other people's money, and contains chapters on:

- procedures
- financial transactions
- responding to financial abuse
- self-employed or directly employed care workers
- security and insurance
- helping service users with their finances
- gifts, wills and bequests
- collecting charges
- service users who are unable to manage their financial affairs.

Written in clear, jargon-free language, the book offers a wealth of information and advice, and contains examples, case studies, relevant care standards, summaries of some recent local government ombudsman cases and a glossary of terms.

£6.99 0-86242-293-0

The Carer's Handbook: What to do and who to turn to

Marina Lewycka

£6.99 0-86242-262-0

Caring for someone who is dying

Penny Mares

£6.99 0-86242-260-4

The Carers Handbook series has been written for the families and friends of older people. It guides readers through key care situations and aims to help readers make informed, practical decisions. All the books in the series:

- are packed full of detailed advice and information
- offer step-by-step guidance on the decisions which need to be taken
- examine all the options available
- are full of practical checklists and case studies
- point you towards specialist help
- guide you through the social services maze
- help you to draft a personal plan of action
- are fully up to date with recent guidelines and issues
- draw on Age Concern's wealth of experience.

Working with Family Carers

Jacqui Wood and Phill Watson

This multi-disciplinary handbook is designed to enable care professionals to view family carers as perhaps their greatest resource and to work in partnership with them. It provides clear and detailed information on every aspect of working with carers, both practically and emotionally. The authors – both experienced practitioners – offer practical tips and experience on topics such as:

- carrying out an assessment
- working with other agencies
- financial difficulties
- emotional and physical stress
- relevant legislation
- ensuring carers' rights.

£14.99 0-86242-230-2

Dementia Care: A handbook for residential and day care

Alan Chapman, Donna Gilmour and Iain McIntosh

This revised edition of a successful book stresses a more holistic approach to the support of people with dementia: in essence, dementia, as an illness, does not rob the person of the influence of their past life. There is now a greater understanding of the experience of dementia for individuals and its impact on families and partners, and working with people with dementia can be challenging. Topics include:

- the individual and their previous lifestyle
- staff teamwork
- approaches to the person
- issues for day care
- what is dementia and what is not?
- health matters
- behaviour as a response to the living environment
- behaviour as a response to the daily routine and staff actions
- dilemmas and challenges
- feelings of loss, pain and palliative care.

Each chapter concludes with suggested training exercises linked to case studies. A comprehensive, practical guide addressing the delivery of care to people with dementia, this book has been designed for use by those working in both residential and day care settings, providing sound advice on good practice and offering reassurance and support.

£14.99 0-86242-313-9

Introducing Dementia

David Sutcliffe

This book is an introductory guide to the whole field of dementia, particularly as it manifests itself in today's society. The book explores:

- the physical process of dementia
- communications
- the effect of dementia on the mind
- financial matters
- the range of major, as well as less common dementias
- the issues of care at home, as well as long-term care.

Stressing the importance of person-centred care, which emphasises physical, emotional, psychological and spiritual care, this book promises to raise awareness and improve standards.

£14.99 0-86242-283-3

If you would like to order any of these titles, please write to the address below, enclosing a cheque or money order for the appropriate amount (plus £1.95 p&p) made payable to Age Concern England. Credit card orders may be made on 0870 44 22 044 (for individuals); 0870 44 22 120 (AC federation, other organisations and institutions). Fax: 0870 44 22 034.

Age Concern Books
PO Box 232
Newton Abbot
Devon TQ12 4XQ

Age Concern Information Line/Factsheets subscription

Age Concern produces 44 comprehensive factsheets designed to answer many of the questions older people (or those advising them) may have. These include money and benefits, health, community care, leisure and education, and housing. For up to five free factsheets, telephone: 0800 00 99 66 (7am–7pm, seven days a week, every day of the year). Alternatively you may prefer to write to Age Concern, FREE-POST (SWB 30375), ASHBURTON, Devon TQ13 7ZZ.

For professionals working with older people, the factsheets are available on an annual subscription service, which includes updates throughout the year. For further details and costs of the subscription, please write to Age Concern at the above Freepost address.

Index